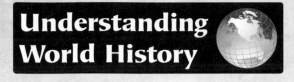

Understanding
World History

# The Black Death

Other titles in the series include:

Ancient Egypt
Ancient Greece
Ancient Rome
The Decade of the 2000s
The Holocaust
The Early Middle Ages
The Late Middle Ages
The Renaissance

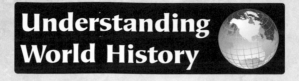

**Understanding World History**

# The Black Death

Stephen Currie

**Bruno Leone**
**Series Consultant**

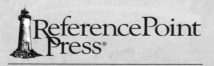

ReferencePoint
Press®

San Diego, CA

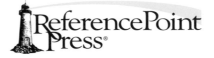

**For more information, contact:**
ReferencePoint Press, Inc.
PO Box 27779
San Diego, CA 92198
www. ReferencePointPress.com

LIBRARY OF CONGRESS CATALOGING-IN-PUBLICATION DATA

Currie, Stephen, 1960-
  The black death / by Stephen Currie.
     p. cm. -- (Understanding world history series)
  Includes bibliographical references and index.
  ISBN-13: 978-1-60152-480-5 (hardback)
  ISBN-10: 1-60152-480-3 (hardback)
  1. Black Death--History. 2. Plague--History I. Title.
  RC171.C87 2013
  614.5'732--dc23
                                                              2012021114

# Contents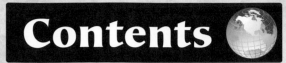

# Foreword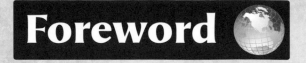

When the Puritans first emigrated from England to America in 1630, they believed that their journey was blessed by a covenant between themselves and God. By the terms of that covenant they agreed to establish a community in the New World dedicated to what they believed was the true Christian faith. God, in turn, would reward their fidelity by making certain that they and their descendants would always experience his protection and enjoy material prosperity. Moreover, the Lord guaranteed that their land would be seen as a shining beacon—or in their words, a "city upon a hill,"—which the rest of the world would view with admiration and respect. By embracing this notion that God could and would shower his favor and special blessings upon them, the Puritans were adopting the providential philosophy of history—meaning that history is the unfolding of a plan established or guided by a higher intelligence.

The concept of intercession by a divine power is only one of many explanations of the driving forces of world history. Historians and philosophers alike have subscribed to numerous other ideas. For example, the ancient Greeks and Romans argued that history is cyclical. Nations and civilizations, according to these ancients of the Western world, rise and fall in unpredictable cycles; the only certainty is that these cycles will persist throughout an endless future. The German historian Oswald Spengler (1880–1936) echoed the ancients to some degree in his controversial study *The Decline of the West*. Spengler asserted that all civilizations inevitably pass through stages comparable to the life span of a person: childhood, youth, adulthood, old age, and, eventually, death. As the title of his work implies, Western civilization is currently entering its final stage.

Joining those who see purpose and direction in history are thinkers who completely reject the idea of meaning or certainty. Rather, they reason that since there are far too many random and unseen factors at work on the earth, historians would be unwise to endorse historical predictability of any type. Warfare (both nuclear and conventional), plagues, earthquakes, tsunamis, meteor showers, and other catastrophic world-changing events have loomed large throughout history and prehistory. In his essay "A Free Man's Worship," philosopher and mathematician Bertrand

Russell (1872–1970) supported this argument, which many refer to as the nihilist or chaos theory of history. According to Russell, history follows no preordained path. Rather, the earth itself and all life on earth resulted from, as Russell describes it, an "accidental collocation of atoms." Based on this premise, he pessimistically concluded that all human achievement will eventually be "buried beneath the debris of a universe in ruins."

Whether history does or does not have an underlying purpose, historians, journalists, and countless others have nonetheless left behind a record of human activity tracing back nearly 6,000 years. From the dawn of the great ancient Near Eastern civilizations of Mesopotamia and Egypt to the modern economic and military behemoths China and the United States, humanity's deeds and misdeeds have been and continue to be monitored and recorded. The distinguished British scholar Arnold Toynbee (1889–1975), in his widely acclaimed twelve-volume work entitled *A Study of History,* studied twenty-one different civilizations that have passed through history's pages. He noted with certainty that others would follow.

In the final analysis, the academic and journalistic worlds mostly regard history as a record and explanation of past events. From a more practical perspective, history represents a sequence of building blocks—cultural, technological, military, and political—ready to be utilized and enhanced or maligned and perverted by the present. What that means is that all societies—whether advanced civilizations or preliterate tribal cultures—leave a legacy for succeeding generations to either embrace or disregard.

Recognizing the richness and fullness of history, the ReferencePoint Press Understanding World History series fosters an evaluation and interpretation of history and its influence on later generations. Each volume in the series approaches its subject chronologically and topically, with specific focus on nations, periods, or pivotal events. Primary and secondary source quotations are included, along with complete source notes and suggestions for further research.

Moreover, the series reflects the truism that the key to understanding the present frequently lies in the past. With that in mind, each series title concludes with a legacy chapter that highlights the bonds between past and present and, more important, demonstrates that world history is a continuum of peoples and ideas, sometimes hidden but there nonetheless, waiting to be discovered by those who choose to look.

# Important Events During the Time of the Black Death

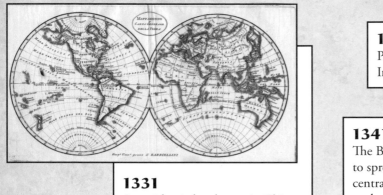

**1331**
An epidemic breaks out in China; possibly the Black Death.

**1345**
Plague reaches India and Iran, killing millions.

**1341**
The Black Death begins to spread outward from central Asia, following trade routes.

| 1330 | 1335 | 1340 | 1345 |
| --- | --- | --- | --- |

**1330**
The Black Death probably appears in central Asia.

**1339**
An epidemic, possibly the Black Death, appears in Kyrgyzstan.

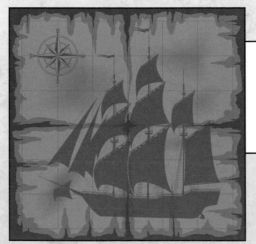

**1346–1347**
Plague reaches Kaffa and is transported to Messina, Sicily, by Genoese sailors; it spreads across Sicily and reaches mainland Italy.

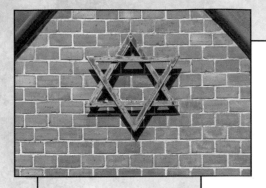

**1348**

The Black Death infects Italy, France, Spain, and the Netherlands, along with parts of Germany and England; Europe's Jews are accused of creating and spreading the plague; persecution of Jews begins.

**1351**

The Black Death arrives in Russia and begins to die out in much of western Europe.

| 1348 | 1349 | 1350 | 1351 / 1361 |

**1349**

Attacks on Jews reach their highest level; plague spreads through the rest of central Europe and into eastern Europe.

**1361**

Another outbreak of plague begins in western Europe.

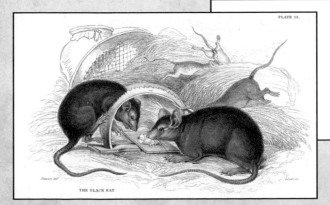

PLATE 25.

THE BLACK RAT.

**1350**

Italian writer Giovanni Boccaccio begins writing *The Decameron,* a fictional book about the plague that includes a famous real-life description of the plague in Florence, Italy.

# The Defining Characteristics of the Black Death

During the middle of the 1300s, a terrible disease known as the Black Death swept across much of the eastern hemisphere. Spreading eventually from China in the east to Iceland in the west, the disease left behind a trail of unspeakable devastation. Between 1347 and 1350, in particular, the Black Death sickened about half of Europe's total population, along with many millions more in Asia and northern Africa. Those who contracted the disease—which most historians and medical experts today identify as a rodent- and insect-borne infection called the plague—developed nasty purple swellings, dangerously high fevers, intense pain, and violent, bloody coughs. Though some victims of the disease did manage to recover, most did not. "A third of the world died,"[1] mourned Jean Froissart, a French chronicler of the time.

By any standard, the Black Death was a disaster of appalling proportions. The number of deaths alone was overwhelming. Modern estimates of the worldwide death toll range from 50 million to 125 million; some historians suspect that the actual number may be higher still. Hundreds of years after it ended, the Black Death remains the deadliest epidemic in world history—and no other epidemic has come close. Indeed, the Black Death stands as one of the most lethal catastrophes of any kind ever recorded. The intense sufferings of most of the plague's victims, moreover, added considerably to the horror of the pestilence. As a rule, death came to the infected only after several days and nights of terrible pain, confusion, and emotional distress. One observer, for example, noted the "sputum [mucus] suffused with blood" and the "disgusting and stinking breath" of many of the victims. "The throat and tongue . . . were black and congested with blood,"[2] the writer added.

Nor was the suffering during the years of the Black Death limited to those who actually caught the disease. Nearly every survivor lost multiple family members, neighbors, and friends to the pestilence. No one knew, moreover, when the plague would strike next. People went to bed each night wondering whether their husband, wife, or child would wake up the next morning with the high fever and the swellings that signified the onset of the illness. Life in the time of the Black Death was uncertain and fragile, and that uncertainty and fragility produced great stress. As historian John Aberth writes, "Imagine that, tomorrow or the next day, every other person you see around you may be dead, and you may grasp something of the terror that this disease could inspire."[3]

In many cases, in fact, deaths were so common and grief so paralyzing that society came close to breaking down altogether. With hundreds of people dying every day in some European cities, gravediggers could not keep up with the growing pile of corpses. The dead, an Italian writer observed, had to be stacked "layer upon layer just like one puts layers of cheese on lasagna."[4] The supply of laborers, priests, and notaries dwindled sharply in some places, making even the simplest of tasks almost impossible to accomplish. Trade ground almost to a halt, business transactions were delayed for months, and the deaths of farmers led to severely diminished harvests. "No one knew where to turn for help,"[5] noted a chronicler in a part of England where the death toll among peasants was especially high.

## Emotion, Sorrow, and Hope

Far worse than unburied corpses or meager harvests, however, was the Black Death's ability to cut the emotional ties that connected one person to another. Terrified of catching the disease themselves, people throughout the affected areas of the globe abandoned their responsibilities to the sick and the dying. Many priests and physicians—professionals responsible for serving those in need—fled their plague-stricken communities in an effort to save themselves, leaving the afflicted behind. And in a shocking number of cases, the sick were abandoned even by their own families. "Brother was forsaken by brother, oftentimes husband by wife," wrote Italian author Giovanni Boccaccio. "Fathers and mothers were found to abandon their own children to their fate, untended, unvisited as if they had been strangers."[6]

There is no defending the actions of the survivors who abandoned their loved ones to suffering and death. Still, given the horrors of the plague, it is understandable that people sometimes responded to it in ways that were considerably less than heroic. Even the finest minds of

*The Black Death, the deadliest epidemic the world has ever known, brought physical suffering and emotional torment to fourteenth-century Europe. An engraving depicts the terrible toll of the disease on residents of Florence, Italy, in the mid-1300s.*

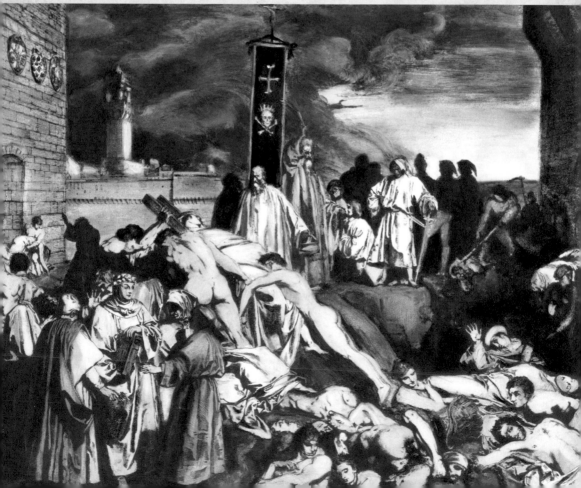

the era were at a loss to explain the Black Death, much less to contain it. Its randomness, its virulence, its staying power—all were beyond the experience of fourteenth-century Europeans. Certainly the Black Death represented suffering on an unimaginable scale. Worse, nothing seemed able to stop its progress. "All the wisdom and ingenuity of man were unavailing,"[7] lamented a chronicler.

In the end, the Black Death lasted only about four years before vanishing in the early 1350s. Though it returned to Europe on several occasions over the next few centuries, it never again approached the intensity and severity that characterized it between 1347 and 1351. Although the worst of the Black Death came and went in a relatively short time, the epidemic of the 1340s changed Europe forever. The Black Death was a time of deep despair, when it seemed that civilization was crumbling, God was absent, and the assumptions people held about the world were no longer valid. As an Italian observer wrote in 1348, as the Black Death was killing more than half the people of his town, "I can't go on. Everywhere one turns there is death and bitterness."[8] The story of the Black Death is one about the triumph of fear and sorrow—and the loss of hope.

# Chapter 1

# What Conditions Led to the Black Death?

The Black Death appeared in Europe toward the end of the medieval period, or the Middle Ages, an era that lasted from approximately the fifth century to the late fourteenth. The medieval period was a difficult time in European history, and the 1300s were no exception. Most Europeans of the time were peasants, desperately poor tenant farmers who struggled year after year to make ends meet. With famine, war, and disease all too common, mortality rates were extremely high: the average rural European of the early 1300s lived less than thirty years, and death tolls in the continent's crowded, trash-strewn cities were often even higher. The continent was ruled by kings, nobles, and bishops who often ignored the needs of their people and enriched themselves at the expense of the poor. Few people could read and write, modern scientific thinking was nonexistent, and most Europeans had little or no knowledge of the world beyond their own communities.

When the Black Death reached Europe in the late 1340s, it came to a society that was in many ways an ideal breeding ground for a plague. The weakened state of the rural population, the filth that littered the cities, the widespread ignorance of science and the outside world—the late medieval world was a place where the Black Death could easily thrive. Even one of medieval Europe's few successes—a steady rise in trade that marked the late 1200s and early 1300s—helped the pestilence gain a foothold in Europe and spread throughout the population. Many conditions, then—both positive and negative—allowed it to enter the continent and to flourish once it arrived.

## Hunger

Of all the features that characterized life in medieval Europe, one of the most consistent was hunger. Even in a temperate summer, peasants across the continent had difficulty raising enough food to feed their families. Much of Europe's farmland was marginal, its soil too low in nutrients to allow it to produce a reliably decent crop. Neither were all summers temperate ones. Cold, wet weather flooded fields, stunted crops, and led to severely diminished harvests. Hot, dry summers, in turn, caused droughts that shriveled crops soon after they began to grow, again dropping harvest levels well below what most farmers could bear. To make matters worse, the lands were usually owned not by the peasants themselves but by noblemen who demanded a portion of each farmer's crop as a form of rent. This system, known as feudalism, made it even more difficult for farmers to harvest enough to feed their families.

In some cases the combination of marginal farmland, bad weather, and excessive rents resulted in widespread starvation and death. Throughout most of Europe, rain fell almost constantly during the growing seasons of 1315 and 1316, for example, and the resulting loss of crops led directly to the deaths of hundreds of thousands of people, perhaps more. "Nor does anyone remember so much dearth and famine to have prevailed in the past," wrote English chronicler John de Trokelowe, "nor so much mortality to have attended it."[9] Stories of the time described people scavenging for spoiled meat and rotting grain; a few even claimed that people resorted to cannibalism, though many historians reject these tales as exaggerations. Nonetheless, there is no question that death from starvation was a very real occurrence in the first part of the 1300s.

Most European peasants of the time, to be sure, did not die when harvests were bad. Somehow or other, even in the leanest years, they

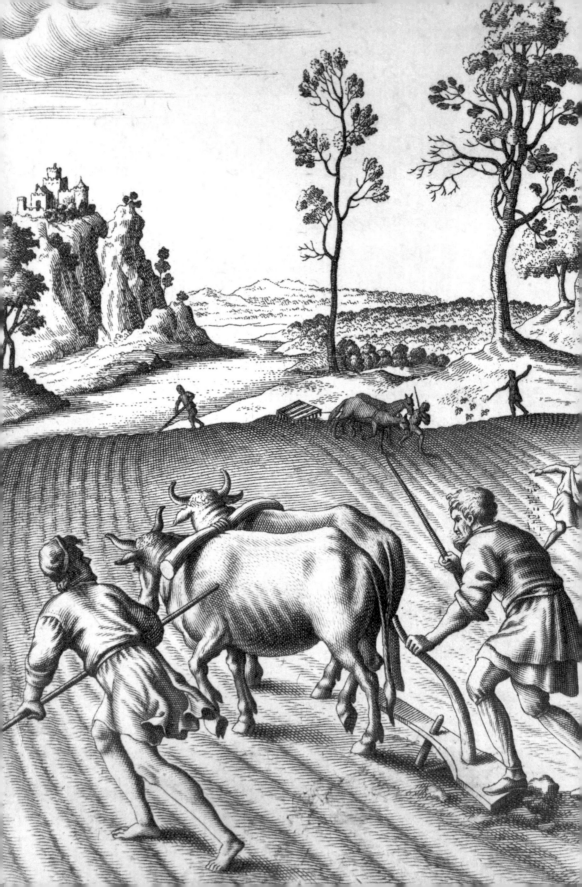

*Peasant farmers plow a strip of land in hopes of a bountiful harvest. More often than not, crops died from flooding or drought. Even in good years, marginal farmland yielded a meager harvest, and much of what did grow had to be given in payment to the landowner.*

managed to find sufficient food to keep them alive. But the cumulative effect of poor harvests had an effect. A steady deficiency of calories, vitamins, and nutrients weakened bones, depleted energy levels, and stunted growth. Those who never had quite enough to eat became increasingly vulnerable to infections of all kinds. Almost any contagious illness could kill when it arrived in a region where hunger was prevalent. "The one who is poorly nourished by unsubstantial food," noted French writer Simon de Couvin following one such outbreak, "fell victim to the merest breath of . . . disease."[10] Existing records support de Couvin's contention; death rates from infection did tend to be higher in places where poor harvests were frequent.

Europe's difficulty feeding its people thus contributed significantly to the horrors of the Black Death. A large percentage of Europeans were chronically hungry and weak, making them especially defenseless against the ravages of the Black Death. To be sure, the plague killed plenty of people who were vigorous and well fed, but it did its deadliest work among those whose health was already compromised owing to lack of food. A healthier society, one able to provide sufficient food to all its members, might well have experienced a much lower death toll from the Black Death than did medieval Europe.

## "Drowning in Filth"

In addition to lingering and widespread hunger, medieval Europe was also characterized by poor sanitation. People of the fourteenth century, to put it bluntly, did not value cleanliness. Very few Europeans of the time paid much attention to personal hygiene. The poor usually did not own enough clothes to make frequent clothing changes practical, and all but the extremely rich often wore the same clothing for many days in a row. Washing the body with soap and water, moreover, was frowned upon as a needless indulgence at best, a sin at worst. "To those who are well, and especially to the young," thundered St. Benedict, an influential church leader of the early Middle Ages, "bathing shall seldom be permitted."[11] As a result of these policies, historian John Aberth writes, most medieval Europeans "hosted a microscopic zoo . . . on their bodies as well as in their clothes."[12]

Nor was personal hygiene the only issue. Both the urban and rural poor lived in conditions so squalid and unhygienic that even regular bathing might not have made much difference. Most peasants lived in ramshackle huts with wooden walls held together by dried mud and roofs made from straw, hay, or grass. Inside the huts air circulated poorly if at all. Insects, mice, and other pests made their homes within the walls, under the floorboards, in the thatch that formed the roof, and in the straw bedding used by most rural Europeans. These creatures were so common, in fact, that a phrasebook of the time taught English travelers how to translate "The fleas bite me so!"[13] into French.

The unhealthy living conditions in rural Europe were not simply the result of poor construction techniques and unsuitable furnishings. Throughout the medieval period many peasants kept domestic animals in their houses—among them cats, dogs, sheep, chickens, and cows. As historian Colin Platt describes it, the traditional arrangement was "animals at one end [of the house] and family at the other."[14] Still, complete separation was not possible given that the limited resources available to most farmers of the time did not permit them to build houses of any significant size. The typical peasant home, then, was loud, chaotic, crowded, smelly, and filled with animal dander and piles of excrement. This was scarcely a recipe for healthy living.

Compared to the towns and cities of the European Middle Ages, though, rural areas were immaculate. As historian John Kelly sums up with only minimal exaggeration, "The medieval city was drowning in filth."[15] There was no municipal trash collection, so people cheerfully tossed their garbage out their windows, filling streets and gutters with rotting vegetables, spoiled meat, and stale bread. Blood from dead and dying animals ran down the streets outside butcher stores. Half-wild

# Pessimism

The deprivation that characterized life in the early 1300s quite naturally affected the way the people of western Europe viewed the world around them. Europeans at the end of the medieval period were a deeply pessimistic people who focused on the hardships of life much more than on its comforts. As they saw it, life was meant to be endured, not enjoyed. Even religion was little comfort to the Europeans of the time. Earthquakes, famine, disease, all manner of disasters were widely interpreted as the judgment of God upon a wicked and ungrateful people. "When God saw that the world was so over proud," wrote a poet in 1327, "He sent a dearth [that is, famine] on earth, and made it full hard." Worse yet, it was commonly accepted that God's antagonism toward humanity would continue after death. According to the theology of the time, only a small number of Christians would go to heaven; the rest would be damned to hell for all eternity.

Quoted in John Aberth, *From the Brink of Apocalypse.* New York: Routledge, 2000.

dogs and pigs roamed the cities, leaving droppings everywhere. Human waste was a problem too. Most city residents used communal latrines, which produced unbearable smells and attracted rats and other vermin. Those unwilling or unable to make the trip to the latrines filled up containers called chamber pots in the privacy of their own rooms and then dumped the contents out the window and into the street below.

Just as the lack of hygiene in the countryside brought trouble to rural Europeans, the lack of sanitation in medieval European cities presented significant problems for urban residents. Drinking water in towns and cities came largely from local rivers—but with these waterways fouled by animal and human waste, they carried pathogens that

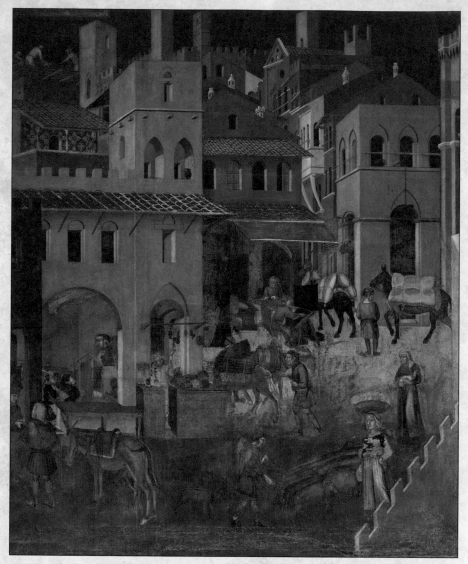

*Discarded, rotting, and spoiled food; blood from butchered animals; and human and animal waste polluted the streets and gutters of medieval Europe's crowded cities. Germs and disease spread freely in these conditions. Pictured is a typical medieval street scene in Italy.*

could make people extremely sick. Garbage, animal droppings, and blood attracted pests of all descriptions; these included rodents, such as rats and mice, and insects like mosquitoes and houseflies. Most historians agree that the unhealthy conditions in medieval towns and cities killed even more people than the lack of cleanliness among peasants. "Medieval urban Europe [was] so disease-ridden," writes Kelly, "no city of any size could maintain its population without a constant influx of immigrants from the countryside."[16]

## Misunderstanding Disease

Another cause of the Black Death in Europe was a general ignorance of what disease was and how it was transmitted. By today's standards, medical knowledge during the Middle Ages was almost nonexistent. To be fair, that was not the fault of doctors or other healers. Modern science recognizes that disease is caused by bacteria, viruses, and other pathogens far too small to be seen; this principle is known as germ theory. But the medieval era ended many years before the invention of the microscope, which made it possible to see these tiny organisms, and several centuries before scientists first proposed germ theory. Medieval Europeans would have scoffed at the notion that invisible objects floated through the air and the water, infecting people who breathed them in or drank them. Unfortunately, because disease was spread in exactly this way, the healers of the medieval period were unable to do much to prevent disease from striking their communities or to cure it when it did.

In the absence of germ theory, doctors of the medieval era relied on other principles to explain disease. Chief among these was the theory of the four humors. (Despite the name, these humors had nothing to do with comedy; in this case, the word means "distinctive features.") The theory was drawn from the thinking of the ancient Greeks. Early Greek doctors noted the presence of four liquid substances in every human body: blood; phlegm, or the mucus that forms in the respiratory system; and black bile and yellow bile, fluids that aid in digestion. In part because ancient Greek philosophy valued equilibrium and order, doctors came to see illness as being caused by an imbalance in these four humors. As the Greek physician Hippocrates wrote, "Health is primarily that state in which [the humors] are in correct proportion to each other, both in strength and in quality."[17]

As believers in the four humors theory saw it, the delicate balance between the humors could be destroyed in several ways. Breathing air that was excessively hot and humid, for example, was believed to increase some of the humors at the expense of others and to make people sick. Likewise, doctors agreed that poor diet could throw off the balance. In particular, medieval physicians attributed dozens of symptoms, from hacking coughs to high fevers, to the pernicious effects of an excess of blood. To reduce the blood supply and bring the humors back into balance, doctors bled patients by cutting into veins or by placing blood-sucking leeches on the patient's body. In many cases the process of bloodletting continued until the patient had lost so much blood that he or she fainted. Bloodletting rarely, if ever, did much to cure anyone, but by further weakening the sick, the practice surely worsened the condition of thousands of patients during medieval times—and very likely killed thousands more.

In addition to relying on the theory of humors, medieval medicine rested on several other shaky foundations. One was the notion of bad air. Physicians of the time were convinced that natural disasters, notably earthquakes, poisoned the air by filling it with corrupt vapors. A similar assumption involved astrology; many physicians relied heavily on the stars to make diagnoses and determine cures. "He was grounded in astrology," wrote English author Geoffrey Chaucer approvingly about a fictional doctor who chose "the proper hour for application" of medicines according to "the planets' best position."[18] Neither astrology nor the doctrine of bad air had any kind of objective evidence to back it up. Still, like the theory of humors, these notions were used by physicians throughout medieval Europe. As much as any other factor, the sorry state of European medical knowledge during the mid-1300s was instrumental in bringing about the Black Death.

## Commerce

An ignorance of the basics of medicine, poor sanitation, and widespread hunger were deep-rooted problems in medieval society. And though each of them helped to bring about the Black Death, they made life

# Power in Medieval Europe

**P**ower in fourteenth-century Europe was divided between two distinct groups. One consisted of kings, princes, and other lords. Some of these leaders governed only small territories; the lords who collected rents from tenant farmers fell into this category. Other nobles, however, ruled over regions where tens of thousands of people lived, and a handful controlled entire nations. Edward III, for example, was king of England from 1327 to 1377, during which time he transformed England into a formidable military power. Another fourteenth-century king, Louis IV, ruled much of Germany; a third ruler, Philip VI, was king of France. For the most part, these monarchs were autocrats who governed largely as they pleased.

The supremacy of the monarchs and lords was rivaled only by religious leaders. Christianity was divided at the time into two sects. The Orthodox Church was dominant in eastern Europe, and the Western, or Roman Catholic, Church held the allegiance of nearly all western Europeans. The pope, also known as the Bishop of Rome, was the single most powerful religious leader in western Europe during the medieval period, but other bishops had authority too. Much of this power was moral: church leaders determined how Christians had to behave on the earth to reach heaven after death. But the church's power was temporal, or worldly, as well. The Western Church owned a great deal of land, controlled enormous sums of money, and wielded tremendous influence in the nonreligious matters of the time. Together, the church and the nobles accounted for virtually all power in fourteenth-century Europe.

miserable for millions of Europeans long before the plague ever arrived on the continent. The same was not true, however, of increased commerce, another factor that contributed to the plague. Far from causing more pain and suffering, the rise of trade actually boosted the standard of living during the later Middle Ages. Culturally and economically, Europeans were better off with this rise than they would have been without it. Yet the Black Death would not have been nearly so catastrophic—and might never have taken place at all—if not for the growth of trade. The increased commerce of the 1300s, then, was at once beneficial and disastrous, thus representing one of history's great ironies.

Because of the relative poverty of Europe through most of the Middle Ages, medieval Europeans carried on little trade until the 1200s. Europeans had few goods that anyone else wanted, and they could not afford to bring in many materials from outside the continent. In the early 1200s, however, leaders in several Italian city-states set out to establish their communities as important trading centers within the Mediterranean region. By the late 1200s Italian ships were making voyages to places like Egypt, Turkey, and Spain to buy and sell silks and cinnamon, jewels and slaves, wool and timber, and much more. These ventures paid off. As historian William J. Bernstein writes, "A hundred pounds of nutmeg, purchased in medieval Alexandria [a city in Egypt] for ten ducats, might easily go for thirty or fifty ducats on the wharves of Venice."[19] The profits allowed merchants and investors to build more ships and to make more extensive voyages. By the late 1200s Italian ships had journeyed into the Black Sea, east of the Mediterranean; by 1300 they were sailing up Europe's Atlantic coastline as well.

Following the Italians' lead, other European countries soon began to increase their own merchant activities. Several German cities formed a loose confederation known as the Hanseatic League, which was designed to encourage trade in north-central Europe. Farther west, England developed a close commercial relationship with the region known as Flanders, now divided among Belgium and the Netherlands. As an English writer of the early 1300s crowed, "All the nations of the world are kept warm by the wool of England made into cloth by the men of Flanders."[20] By 1340 trade routes had sprung up throughout the continent and beyond—some crisscrossing the seas, some following paths across land, still others making their way along Europe's rivers. Commerce in western Europe during the mid-1300s was greater in both volume and importance than it had been for a thousand years.

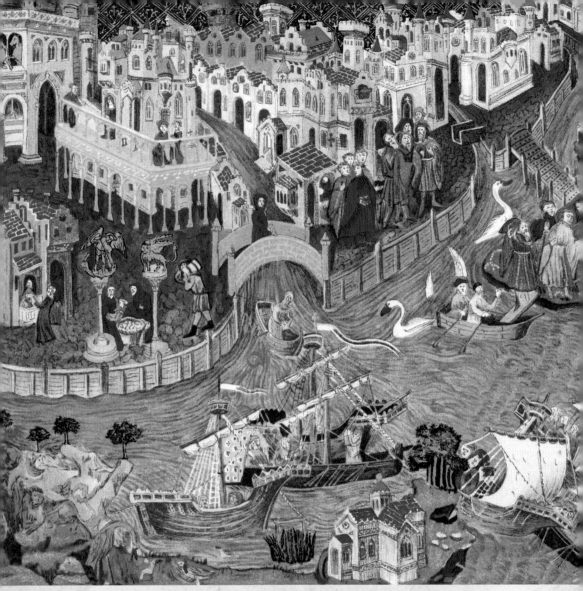

*Merchant and explorer Marco Polo sets out from Venice, Italy, for the Far East in 1271, as depicted in this fourteenth-century illustration. A brisk trade in spices, jewels, fabrics, and more helped to establish Italian city-states as important trading centers—and as key points in the spread of the plague.*

The rise of commerce at the end of the Middle Ages was unquestionably of great benefit to many Europeans. Spices, jewels, fabrics, and other materials that could not be produced within Europe improved the quality of life for those who were already well off and could afford to buy luxurious goods. Merchants became wealthy as trade grew in importance, and the nobles and clergy who taxed the merchants' fortunes profited as well. Even Europe's poor benefitted. The market for woolen cloth, for example, provided jobs for the people of Flanders, and Italian sailors found their services increasingly in demand as merchant fleets grew in size.

## Trade Routes and the Plague

But not everything that moved along the trade routes of the 1200s and the early 1300s was good for the people of Europe. By linking European communities so closely, trade ultimately made the continent more vulnerable. Along with spawning positive changes, the growing commerce of late medieval Europe also ushered in something that would prove disastrous: the microbe that caused the Black Death. Though the traders of the 1300s had no way of knowing it, the ships and caravans that carried spices from the Black Sea to Barcelona, silks from Cairo to Cologne, and timber from Lübeck to London simultaneously brought in the virus that would cause one of the worst disasters in history.

The conditions that led to the Black Death, then, were of two very different kinds. On the one hand, the epidemic stemmed directly from the aspects of medieval life that stressed the population even before the arrival of the plague. Without the poor hygiene, the food shortages, and the ignorance of disease that marked the late medieval era, the Black Death might never have been able to devastate Europe. But on the other hand, the epidemic was also made possible by one of the few activities that brought income and a sense of pride to late medieval Europe. If not for the growing trade networks of the 1300s, the plague might never have arrived in Europe, let alone spread any significant distance. In this way an unusual combination of positives and negatives combined to unleash the Black Death on the unsuspecting citizens of the late Middle Ages.

# Chapter 2

# The Black Death Arrives

**S**ometime during the 1320s or early 1330s a mysterious and alarming disease began to affect the people of central Asia. In 1331, for example, records show that an epidemic took root in a western Chinese province, wiping out large swaths of the population in a matter of weeks. The disease appeared again a year or two later, this time in Mongolia. Before long it infiltrated sections of Russia as well. By 1339, when a large number of people in what is now Kyrgyzstan died of the disease, the infection had been named. "This is the grave of Kutluk," reads a tombstone in a Kyrgyz cemetery. "He died of the plague with his wife Magnu-Kelka."[21]

Whether the disease that swept through central Asia in the 1330s was actually the Black Death is a subject of some debate among historians and medical experts. The few chronicles that survive from the period are generally vague about the symptoms of the epidemics, so it is difficult to be sure that those who became sick experienced the swellings, headaches, fevers, and coughs associated with the Black Death. Even the inscription on the gravestone in Kyrgyzstan may not be enough to identify the 1339 epidemic as the Black Death. Some experts believe that the word translated as *plague* was used to describe other illnesses in that time and place as well.

Still, there are good reasons to believe that the epidemics of the 1330s were the first appearances of the Black Death. One of these reasons involves the connection of central Asia to the microorganism that causes the plague. This microorganism, known as *Yersinia pestis* (the bacillus was first identified in the 1890s by Swiss scientist Alexandre

Yersin), or *Y. pestis,* most commonly circulates among rodents, especially large rodents like marmots, ground squirrels, and the tarabagan, a burrowing animal about the size of a cat. All of these rodents are native to central Asia—indeed, the tarabagan lives nowhere else. Because of the tendency of central Asian rodents to be infected with the plague bacillus, many scientists have concluded that the region represents ground zero for the Black Death. As one twentieth-century scientist wrote, the rodent population of central Asia made the area the equivalent of "a heap of embers where plague smolders continuously and from which sparks of infection may jump out . . . to set up conflagrations [large fires]."[22]

No matter how widespread the plague bacillus was among the rodent population of central Asia, however, the disease still had to be transmitted to humans. That was not an easy process. Though *Y. pestis* can sometimes be diffused short distances through the air, it usually dies quickly once it leaves the bloodstream of an infected animal. Ground squirrels, marmots, and most other large central Asian rodents make their homes in rugged, mountainous areas and avoid humans whenever possible. Since few humans ever come into direct contact with a marmot or a tarabagan, it is nearly impossible for *Y. pestis* to move directly from these creatures to people. However, scientists know that transmission is much more likely if two other animal species are included in the chain—and historians believe that this is precisely what happened in the years around 1330.

## Enter the Rat

The first link in the chain is the rat. Small, quick, and willing to eat almost anything, rats can be found almost everywhere on the globe, and central Asia is no exception. During the 1320s or early 1330s, experts theorize, a rat in a region near Mongolia or Kyrgyzstan came into contact with a tarabagan or marmot that was carrying *Y. pestis.* Perhaps the carrier bit the rat in a fight over territory or food. Alternatively, the rat might have fed on the larger animal's corpse. Either way, the encounter allowed the *Y. pestis* bacillus to enter the rat's bloodstream.

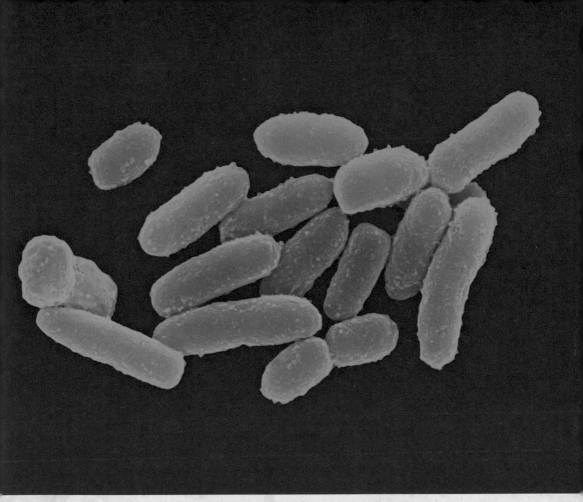

Yersinia pestis *(pictured in a colored scanning electron micrograph) is the microorganism that causes bubonic plague. In the Middle Ages it was transmitted to humans primarily by fleas that had bitten infected rats.*

The transfer of *Y. pestis* to the rat was an essential first step in the spreading of the Black Death. In stark contrast to marmots and ground squirrels, the rat does not avoid people. On the contrary, rats frequently choose to live as close to people as possible so they can steal the food grown, prepared, and stored by their unwilling human hosts. The connection between rats and humanity is as old as history. As long ago as the tenth century BC, for example, people in India routinely prayed for relief from rat infestations. "Kill the burrowing rodents which devastate our food grains," reads a supplication from the period. "Slice their hearts, break their necks, plug their mouths, so that they cannot destroy our food."[23]

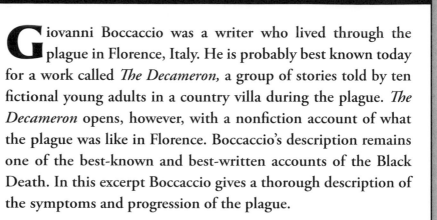

Giovanni Boccaccio was a writer who lived through the plague in Florence, Italy. He is probably best known today for a work called *The Decameron,* a group of stories told by ten fictional young adults in a country villa during the plague. *The Decameron* opens, however, with a nonfiction account of what the plague was like in Florence. Boccaccio's description remains one of the best-known and best-written accounts of the Black Death. In this excerpt Boccaccio gives a thorough description of the symptoms and progression of the plague.

> At the onset of the disease both men and women were afflicted by a sort of swelling in the groin or under the armpits which sometimes attained the size of a common apple or egg. Some of these swellings were larger and some smaller, and were commonly called boils. From these two starting points the boils began in a little while to spread and appear generally all over the body. Afterwards, the manifestation of the disease changed into black or livid spots on the arms, thighs, and the whole person. In many these blotches were large and far apart, in others small and closely clustered. Like the boils, which had been and continued to be a certain indication of coming death, these blotches had the same meaning for everyone on whom they appeared [that is, impending death]. . . . Not only did few recover, but on the contrary almost everyone died within three days of the appearance of the signs—some sooner, some later.

Quoted in Jackson J. Spielvogel, *Western Civilization Volume A: To 1500.* Farmington Hills, MI: Cengage Learning, 2008, p. 306.

A rat that was infected with *Y. pestis*, then, was far more likely than a marmot or a ground squirrel to bring the plague bacillus into close contact with humans. Still, the chain was not complete. To actually infect a human being, *Y. pestis* needs a way to make the jump from the body of a carrier rat into a person's bloodstream. That can happen if a rat bites or scratches a human, but rat attacks on people have never been common. It strains belief to imagine that even a tiny percentage of those who died from the Black Death suffered a rat bite in the weeks before succumbing to the illness.

Therefore, spreading the contagion to people usually required a second link in the chain: the flea. Like rats, fleas have been humanity's constant companions since the beginning of time. But unlike rats, which compete with humans for food, fleas feed directly off the blood of humans and other animals. When a flea sucks the blood of an infected rat, it picks up the *Y. pestis* bacillus from the rat's bloodstream. If it then bites another rat, it transfers the infection to the second rat. And if it bites a human, the disease moves into the victim's bloodstream. "As many as one hundred thousand bacilli can be injected into a [mammal] by a flea,"[24] writes author Robert Sullivan.

The chain of events that created the Black Death was now forged. Marmots and tarabagans in the central Asian wilderness transmitted the disease to rats, which brought it into close contact with humans; next, fleas bit the infected rats and passed the disease on to humans. Whether the sequence was under way in the early 1330s, as records of central Asian epidemics seem to suggest, or whether it did not actually get its start until later, as some modern experts believe, the process had certainly begun by 1341 at the latest. By this time the plague had successfully made the jump to rats and fleas—and to people. The Black Death had become a full-fledged epidemic.

## Spreading Through Asia

At first the plague did not move far from its point of origin. For several years it remained restricted to the towns and villages of central Asia, attracting little notice elsewhere. In about 1343, however, something changed—scientists are not sure what—and the plague began to spread through much of the rest of Asia. In particular, the contagion moved south to India, east into central China, and west toward Iran and Turkey, traveling at an average speed of several miles a day. The Black Death was on the move.

Wherever the Black Death went in Asia, it followed well-traveled trade routes. That was no coincidence. Though rats and fleas rarely travel far on their own, they can cover much greater distances when concealed in the wagons of a trading caravan. As historian William J. Bernstein writes, "Plague is a disease of trade."[25] The most common way of spreading the plague, then, involved the trade wagons and carts that belonged to the merchants of Asia. First, infected rats, together with the fleas they carried, climbed aboard a merchant's wagon when it stopped in Mongolia or Kyrgyzstan. Then, somewhere down the road, the rats and their attendant fleas left the wagon and spread the contagion to another community. The process repeated itself again and again, each time moving the infection farther from its central Asian origins.

It is also possible that the rapid spread of the plague was helped along by the fact that the plague can take on different forms. In its classic form, described previously, the disease is transmitted by rats and fleas and cannot move directly from one person to another. In this form, by far the most common variety, the disease is known as the bubonic plague. But *Y. pestis* also can appear in pneumonic form, which involves transmission of the bacillus through the air. If people infected with the pneumonic plague cough, speak, or even exhale, the plague bacilli infecting their lungs are expelled into the atmosphere. Anyone nearby who inhales the bacilli can become infected too. Pneumonic plague makes it possible for a human being to contract *Y. pestis* without coming into direct contact with a rat or a flea, thus enabling the disease to be transmitted much more quickly.

## Into Europe

By 1346, only about three years after the plague began spreading outward from central Asia, the contagion stretched across much of the

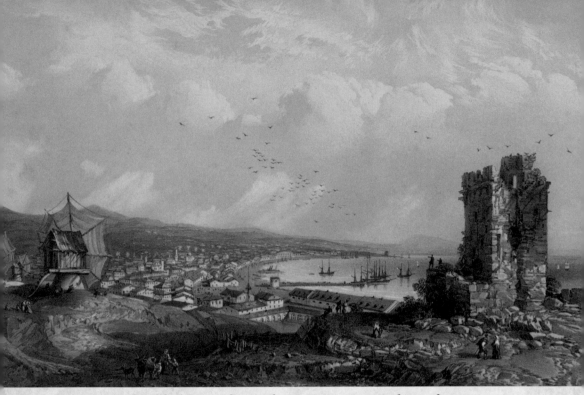

*The town of Kaffa (pictured), on the Crimean Peninsula on the northern coast of the Black Sea, was a major crossroads for traders coming both from the East and the West. As soon as traders realized the extent of contagion in Kaffa, they left—not knowing that they carried infected rats with them wherever they went.*

continent. Wherever it went, it brought devastation. "India was depopulated," wrote one observer. "Mesopotamia [present-day Iraq], Syria, [and] Armenia were covered with dead bodies."[26] By this time word of the growing pestilence had reached Europe. Still, few Europeans showed much concern. In an era when most people never traveled even one hundred miles (161km) from their birthplace, places such as India and Armenia seemed unimaginably distant. What happened in faraway Asia appeared to have no bearing on daily life and work in places like Belgium, Italy, and Poland.

This plague, however, was more powerful and longer lasting than any European suspected. The infection soon made its way into the town of Kaffa on the Crimean Peninsula, a spit of land jutting into the Black Sea. Geographically speaking, Kaffa was a part of Europe. Moreover, it marked the eastern end of an important trade route that joined it to the

# Mortality Rates

Determining the total number of fatalities from the Black Death is extremely difficult. Given the chaos that accompanied the Black Death everywhere it went, no one had the time, energy, or inclination to make an accurate count of the number of dead. Nor was it possible to determine the number of deaths by comparing postplague population records with records from before the plague years. Medieval Europeans seldom tallied population figures, so these records did not exist.

Chroniclers of the time typically overestimated death totals. One writer claimed a death toll of sixty-two thousand in Avignon, France, a figure almost certainly greater than the town's actual population. Boccaccio, similarly, estimated that one hundred thousand died of the plague in Florence. "Who would have thought before the plague that the city held so many inhabitants?" he asked. In reality, it did not; most likely only eighty thousand lived in Florence before the plague arrived.

With accurate records unavailable and eyewitness accounts unreliable, historians have had to estimate mortality rates for the Black Death in a variety of other ways. Most researchers estimate that between 35 and 45 percent of Europe's population died of the pestilence. Europe had between 75 and 100 million inhabitants during the early 1340s, so that implies a death toll in Europe alone of anywhere from about 25 million to 45 million, perhaps considerably higher. Death tolls for Asia and Africa are even more difficult to determine, but modern research suggests that between 50 and 125 million may have died worldwide in the epidemic.

Quoted in Robert S. Gottfried, *The Black Death*. New York: Macmillan, 1983.

Italian city of Genoa, a prominent trading center. The route had been developed in the late 1200s by Genoese merchants, who were attracted to Kaffa because it was connected by road to the wealthier cities of Asia. Thus, it was an excellent place to obtain spices, silks, and other goods not produced in Europe. By the 1340s Kaffa had become a significant crossroads where traders from East and West could meet, mingle, and conduct business.

The Black Death hit Kaffa as it had hit other communities farther east: by wiping out much of the population in just a few months' time. Victims died "as soon as the signs of the disease appeared on their bodies," a chronicler wrote. He noted in particular that the dying developed "swellings in the armpit or groin" and "a putrid fever,"[27] symptoms strongly associated with the plague. Throughout the city people took to their beds with unceasing coughs and terrible headaches; all too often they never got up again. So serious was the outbreak that the leaders of an army trying to take over Kaffa had to call off the attack. Too many of the army's soldiers had died of the disease.

Once they realized the seriousness of the situation, many of the Genoese traders doing business in Kaffa's harbor hurried to load up their goods and sail away. They could not have known it, but they were already too late. Even before the first citizen of Kaffa developed the swellings, headaches, and vomiting characteristic of the Black Death, disease-ridden rats had most likely scurried up the ropes that tied the ships to the docks in Kaffa's harbor. Laden not just with their trade cargo but also with the bacillus that caused the Black Death, the Genoese ships made their way through the Black Sea and into the Mediterranean, heading for home.

## To Sicily

They never arrived. In October 1347 a dozen or so of these ships, probably the remnants of a larger fleet, arrived in the port of Messina on the Mediterranean island of Sicily. An unknown number of the sailors were dead already, and most of the survivors were desperately ill with a disease that no one on the island recognized—but which, to judge from the coughing, the swellings, and the stench of frequent vomiting, was something extremely serious. Moreover, it quickly became apparent that whatever the disease was, it was highly contagious. "The Genoese carried such a disease in their bodies that if anyone so much as spoke with one of them, he was infected with the deadly illness and could not avoid death,"[28] noted Michele da Piazza, an Italian monk. The people of Messina quickly decided that they had made a serious mistake in allowing the Genoese ships to dock in their harbor. Terrified, they forced the Genoese to leave.

But once again, it was already too late. In the reverse of what happened in Kaffa, this time the plague bacillus got off the Genoese ships rather than on them. Whether transmitted by rats and fleas or coughs and sneezes, the Black Death began to spread through the city. Within a matter of days hundreds of people in Messina lay dead and dying, their symptoms exactly the same as those of the Genoese sailors. "A sort of boil . . . the size of a lentil," wrote da Piazza, "erupted on the thigh or the arm, [then] the victims violently coughed up blood, and after three days [of] incessant vomiting . . . they died."[29] The Black Death had gained a foothold in western Europe.

The people of Messina responded to the pestilence in three basic ways—ways that would be repeated again and again during the next several years. One response, of course, was to force the people who brought the disease to leave town. This was a natural and understandable reaction, even if it was not the kindest way to treat the sick. Unfortunately, as the townsfolk quickly realized, evicting the Genoese sailors from the harbor did nothing to prevent the disease from striking. Another response, again quite reasonable, was to run away. Within a few days of the Genoese fleet's arrival, many of Messina's people had abandoned their homes for other parts of the island. Once again, though, the strategy was not very successful. In most cases, those who fled had already been infected by the plague, whether they knew it yet or not.

The third response, appropriate for a deeply Christian society such as medieval Europe, was to turn to religion. Upon recognizing the enormity of the disaster, Messina's surviving leaders immediately contacted officials in the nearby city of Catania. Catania was the proud owner of the bones of St. Agatha of Sicily, a local heroine who had died during the third century; the Roman Catholic Church, the dominant religion in western Europe, considered these bones to be holy. Messina's leaders, hoping that St. Agatha's skeleton could help them defeat the plague, asked to borrow the sacred bones. "If the relics come to Messina," they asserted, "the city will be saved completely from this disease."[30] The Catanians, however, promptly rejected the request. "What a stupid idea on the part of you Messinese," one observer wrote. "Don't you think if [Agatha] wanted to make her home in Messina she would have said so?"[31] In the end the cities compromised: a priest in Catania dipped the bones into a container of holy water and then sent the water on to the people of Messina.

As it turned out, none of the strategies was effective. The plague devastated Messina, killing a third or more of the people despite the presence of the holy water and the expulsion of the Genoese. Those who fled the city do not seem to have survived at any greater rate. Several communities throughout Sicily tried to keep out refugees from Messina and other infected areas, especially if they looked sick. This plan may have helped reduce the incidence of pneumonic plague, but it did nothing to stop the spread of the much more common bubonic variety. As historian Robert S. Gottfried writes, the measure "was designed to exclude people and not the rodents who were plague's principal disseminators."[32] No part of the island was spared as the Black Death swept through urban areas and the countryside alike. Not even Catania was safe. Agatha's bones, it turned out, were not as potent as the Catanians had hoped.

## The Plague Moves On

As the Sicilians died by the thousands, the Genoese fleet that had brought the pestilence to the island sailed off to points unknown. Some sources suggest that the surviving sailors eventually reached Genoa but were forbidden to stay because of their illness. Others say that they split up and made for various ports in Italy and nearby countries. Still another account holds that at least one of the ships sailed toward Gibraltar

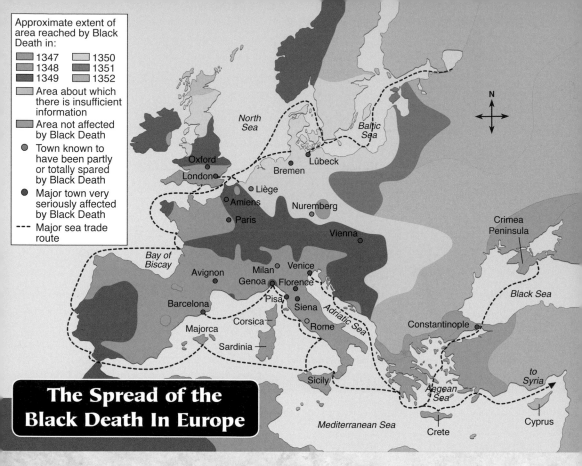

Approximate extent of area reached by Black Death in:
1347
1348
1349
1350
1351
1352
Area about which there is insufficient information
Area not affected by Black Death
● Town known to have been partly or totally spared by Black Death
● Major town very seriously affected by Black Death
--- Major sea trade route

North Sea
Baltic Sea
Oxford
Lûbeck
London
Bremen
Liège
Amiens
Nuremberg
Paris
Vienna
Crimea Peninsula
Bay of Biscay
Milan
Venice
Avignon
Genoa
Florence
Barcelona
Pisa
Siena
Adriatic Sea
Black Sea
Corsica
Rome
Constantinople
Majorca
Sardinia
Sicily
Aegean Sea
to Syria
Mediterranean Sea
Crete
Cyprus

**The Spread of the Black Death In Europe**

at the western end of the Mediterranean. If any of these accounts is true, the continued wanderings of the ships no doubt spread the plague even farther.

But even if the Genoese ships had all sunk immediately upon leaving Messina's harbor, killing every trace of the *Y. pestis* bacilli they were carrying, the rest of western Europe would still have contracted the Black Death. Even as the epidemic continued to rage in the Crimea, Italian trading vessels kept on making their journeys to Kaffa's harbor. Many Italian sea captains and merchants were unwilling to give up their profitable runs to the Black Sea. Not only would suspending operations cost them in the short term, but they worried that rival traders would hurry to Kaffa to fill the gap, thereby costing them in the long term as well. Consequently, ships continued to sail back and forth between disease-infested Kaffa and the still unaffected areas of Italy, and some of these surely carried more than just trade goods. "By November [1347]," writes John Kelly, "there must have been twenty or more plague ships off the southern coast of Europe . . . each armed with the equivalent of a large thermonuclear device."[33]

From its origins in central Asia, the Black Death had taken a dozen or more years to reach Europe. Now, within a matter of weeks, the pestilence had made its way through Sicily, sickening and killing a large percentage of the population. Sicily was a small and relatively unimportant place, but it nonetheless served as an important omen for Europeans beyond its borders. What happened in Messina and Catania could happen in Moscow and Amsterdam, Barcelona and London, Paris and Rome. The Black Death had arrived in Europe, and nothing, it seemed, could stop it.

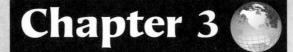

# Chapter 3

# Medicine, Laws, and Prayer

Late in 1347, shortly after the arrival of the Black Death in Sicily, the pestilence reached the European mainland. That December it appeared in Genoa, possibly brought in by the remnants of the fleet that had landed in Sicily, but equally likely by some other trading vessels returning from the Crimea. Like the people of Messina, the Genoese recognized the danger presented by the sick and dying crew members. "[The] ships were driven from the port with burning arrows and other engines of war,"[34] reported chronicler Gabriele de Mussis. But their efforts were too late. Within weeks 30 to 40 percent of Genoa's population was dead.

From Genoa, the Black Death continued to spread. Just as it had in Asia, the plague moved mainly along trade routes. Early in 1348 it attacked Venice, another important trading center on Italy's northeast coast, as well as Marseilles, France, a Mediterranean port west of Genoa. By April the plague had invaded Italian inland cities like Rome and Florence. By the end of the year, moving both by land and by sea, the Black Death had attacked Belgium, Switzerland, Hungary, and Spain, among other countries. It had even jumped across the English Channel to infect southern England.

The plague's progress slowed somewhat during the winter of 1348–1349, but when the weather grew warmer, its pace picked up once again. Ships carried the disease from England to Ireland and along the north German coast. Overland trade routes allowed *Y. pestis* to ravage southern Poland and much of the rest of central Europe. A trading vessel with all its crew dead from the plague drifted into a Norwegian harbor, leading to the infection of Scandinavia. In 1351 the bacillus arrived in Russia, the last significant part of Europe that remained unaffected by the Black Death. In just four years since reaching Messina, the pestilence had conquered the continent.

The effect of the Black Death throughout Europe, moreover, was essentially the same as it had been in Sicily. In some cases it was worse. In Avignon, France, historians believe that half the population died from the Black Death. Hamburg in northern Germany probably lost more than 60 percent of its population, and in Florence, Italy, the death toll was as high as 80 percent. In some smaller communities nearly everyone died. In one Italian monastery that was home to three dozen monks, just one man survived; as historian Barbara Tuchman reports, he "buried the prior [the monastery's leader] and 34 fellow monks one

*A medieval couple suffers from the blisters that signal infection and almost certain death from plague in an illustration that appears in a Swiss manuscript from 1411. Stopping the spread of the Black Death required more knowledge of germs and disease than existed at the time.*

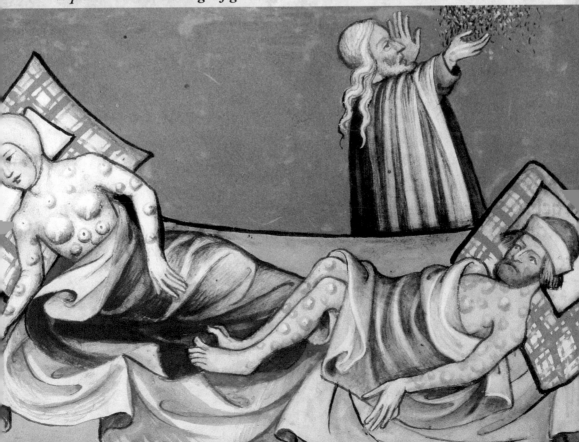

by one, sometimes three a day, until he was left alone with his dog and fled to look for a place that would take him in."[35]

The Black Death represented by far the deadliest threat to Europeans in generations, and something had to be done about it. Many medical, religious, and political leaders throughout Europe turned their entire attention to finding some way to stop the plague's progress and to cure those who were already infected. Most of these attempts were remarkably unsuccessful. Still, in the face of a dreadful and catastrophic epidemic that seemed to have no cure and no end, the people who tried to reverse the course of the illness deserve credit for their efforts. It was far more common, as events proved, for those who were entrusted with caring for the health, lives, and souls of their fellow human beings to do otherwise.

## Medicine and Doctors

With medical knowledge still in its infancy during the late Middle Ages, European doctors had no good scientific explanations that could account for the Black Death. No physician connected the Black Death with the rats and the fleas that infested the continent. "Fleas . . . are not once mentioned in contemporary plague writings," Tuchman points out, "and rats [are mentioned] only incidentally."[36] And although doctors did suspect that the disease could be transmitted directly from one person to another, they had no clear idea how this might be accomplished. Nor were doctors of the time trained to think critically about disease; rather, they relied on the writings of medical practitioners from the classical era, whether those writings made sense or not. Medieval doctors, writes historian John Kelly, had "a typically medieval reverence for authority, especially ancient authority, over observable fact."[37]

In the absence of germ theory, the doctors of the Middle Ages blamed the Black Death on any number of other causes. Many used their astrological expertise to find answers in the stars. At the University of Paris, a group of doctors examined planetary movements and determined that the plague had been caused by the coming together of Mars, Jupiter, and Saturn on March 20, 1345. (They either did not

# Folk Remedies

**P**hysicians during the Middle Ages lived mainly in the cities and the larger towns of Europe. As a result, most medieval farmers and villagers fought disease instead through so-called folk remedies—cures and treatments handed down from one generation to the next. Faced with a fever, an earache, or some other ailment, medieval Europeans could draw from a variety of folk cures.

Many of these remedies were made from plants. Sage, fennel, and coriander, for example, were frequently used in cures. Laurel leaves were often prescribed for stomach complaints. Sometimes the cure called for pounding these plants into a powder and swallowing them. Alternatively, treatments involved boiling the plant and drinking the resulting liquid or draping leaves and roots on the afflicted body part. "Take bean or oat or barley meal," advised a folk treatment for healing wounds without excessive scarring. "Add vinegar and honey, cook together and lay on [the wound] and bind on the sore places."

Other folk remedies involved animals. A folk remedy that claimed to cure shoulder pain, for example, told patients to burn goat hairs and direct the smoke at the affected shoulder. According to another remedy, victims of spider bites could survive if they fried snails, added pepper, and swallowed the result. And a few folk treatments specifically relied on faith. One such cure began by having the patient combine nineteen different plants into a potion, but then it suggested that the patient add holy water and pray.

Quoted in Faith Wallis, *Medieval Medicine: A Reader*. Toronto: University of Toronto Press, 2010, p. 120.

know that the plague had appeared in Asia some years beforehand, or they dismissed that information as irrelevant to the plague in Europe.) "Jupiter, being wet and hot, draws up evil vapors from the earth," the doctors' report explained, "and Mars, because it is immoderately hot and dry, then ignites the vapors."[38] The process caused poisonous materials to form inside the hearts and lungs of many people, though not of everyone.

Other doctors favored an environmental explanation. For years medical experts had associated epidemics with natural disasters, and now they looked back at the historical record in search of unusual events. They soon learned that the coming of the plague to Asia had coincided with several disasters: intense hailstorms, destructive earthquakes, "foul blasts of wind," and a "vast rain of fire."[39] These disasters, commentators agreed, caused bad air to form in the atmosphere; victims of the Black Death then inhaled the air, making them sick. To the experts of the late Middle Ages, the explanation that natural disasters had somehow caused the Black Death seemed as good as any.

## Alternate Explanations

Other doctors accepted the theory of bad air without necessarily agreeing that the trouble was caused by earthquakes or storms. A group of doctors at the University of Montpellier in France, for example, claimed that deadly vapors were primarily to blame for the spread of the plague. This explanation, although not especially scientific, did at least offer a measure of hope to those who had not yet been infected. The Montpellier doctors argued that people could escape the Black Death by staying away from these vapors. According to the doctors, the vapors originated in the south; thus, by shutting or walling off south-facing doors and windows, a family could lower its odds of contracting the disease.

The notion of bad air could also account for the Black Death's ability to transfer itself between people. Doctors of the time sometimes described this process in straightforward terms: plague victims breathed out bad air, and others caught the disease by breathing it in. (This explanation was not all that different from the way pneumonic plague actually works, even though those who championed this theory had no way of knowing how close they were to the cause.) In other explanations, though, the process was more complicated. For example, the Montpellier doctors posited that the deadly vapors, once inhaled by an unwary or south-facing victim, could produce a "toxic spirit" in the body. This spirit could then become visible to others and move from the sick person to a healthy one. "If any well person looks upon that visible spirit," the doctors explained, "he receives the attack of pestilential disease."[40]

The ancient theory of the four humors informed medieval medical thinking about the Black Death, too. In particular, physicians often used this theory to explain why only some people caught the disease. Those whose humors were already out of balance, doctors agreed, were especially likely to succumb. Like the notion that the Black Death was caused by deadly vapors or a toxic spirit, the theory of humors helped medieval Europeans make some sense of the plague. But, of course, it had no scientific validity as an explanation, and applying the theory of the four humors failed to stop the plague or to cure those who were already sick.

## Treatments

Just as doctors had a variety of theories about what caused the Black Death, so, too, did they have a variety of treatments for the disease. And just as the theories typically missed the mark, the treatments also usually left something to be desired. Bleeding, for example, remained a popular cure for plague victims, though it was no more effective for the Black Death than it was for any other malady. Some doctors suggested poking open the swellings on plague sufferers' bodies to let out the pus. Like bleeding, this tactic may have seemed helpful in theory, but in practice it was of no value whatever. Other supposed cures were quite elaborate. One author, for example, recommended that caregivers prepare a potion made from flowers, herbs, "a quantity of good treacle [a syrupy liquid]," some ale, and a roasted egg, then "make the sick drink it for three evenings and three mornings."[41]

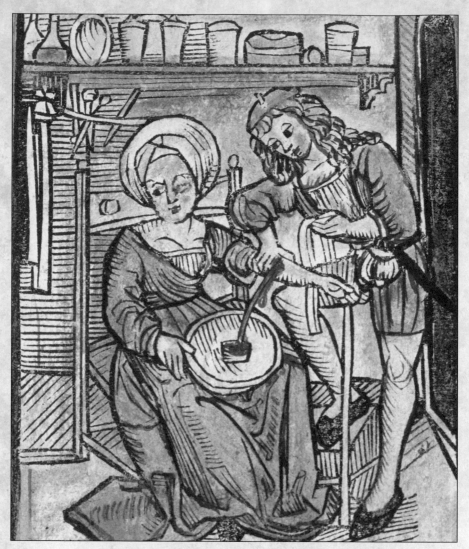

*Bleeding, a popular cure for many diseases of the Middle Ages, had no effect on the course of the plague or other diseases of the time. Some doctors even tried poking open swellings to rid the body of the pus they contained—again to no avail.*

In general, though, doctors of the Black Death era recognized that their cures were useless in the face of the pestilence. Accordingly, doctors' efforts to defeat the Black Death focused more on prevention than on cure. As with the cures, few of these suggestions were especially helpful. Some physicians suggested that people should bury their noses and mouths in sweet-smelling flowers wherever they went, using the aroma to block bad air from entering the body. Similarly, doctors often cautioned people to avoid swampy places where hot and humid air was common.

A competing idea, however, held exactly the opposite course of action. In order to avoid plague, this theory ran, people should expose themselves to odors even more foul than those that brought the Black Death. Thousands of people throughout Europe, taking this advice to heart, bathed in urine or sat for hours in outhouses. "One of the most surreal images to emerge from the Black Death," writes Kelly, "is of knots of people crouched at the edge of municipal latrines inhaling the noxious fumes."[42] The prevailing medical theory that mysterious vapors could cause disease made these recommendations at least somewhat plausible. But none of these treatments could prevent the Black Death.

Other suggestions for warding off the plague focused on diet. Most doctors recommended that people eat plenty of bread and drink plenty of wine, and many urged people to roast their food rather than boil it. Other recommendations were open to more debate. Some physicians advised their patients to eat lamb, cheese, or pomegranates, while others told patients to avoid some or all of these foods. Cabbage, milk, and fish appeared on the must-eat lists of some physicians but on the banned lists of others. In general, though, what people ate had no effect on whether they became ill with the plague—except to the extent that a nutritious diet is generally correlated with good health.

One recommendation that actually did have some success involved fire. Italian physician Gentile da Foligno was one of several doctors to suggest that communities kindle bonfires to ward off the plague. His reasoning was that the heat of the fire would burn the bad vapors out of the air before they could infect people. The reasoning was wrong, of course, but the strategy worked because roaring fires made the area too hot for fleas. Guy de Chauliac, the personal physician of Pope Clement VI, used the same basic tactic, recommending that the pope spend his time sitting between two large fires. Though the fires probably gave Clement some serious discomfort during the summer months, they did keep him from catching the Black Death.

# Caring for the Sick

Even before the plague, members of the medieval medical profession were not held in great regard. Doctors were often viewed as arrogant and overconfident, and some charged them with incompetence as well. A satirical English poem written a generation or so before the Black Death featured a doctor who haughtily tells a woman that of course he can save her sick husband's life; though in truth, the poet points out, the doctor "knows no more than a goose whether [the patient] will live or die."[43] During the plague the reputation of doctors diminished further. Not only were they unable to cure the afflicted, but they also often gave up caring for the sick altogether once it became clear that the patients would not survive. De Chauliac, who did continue to work with the sick, wrote afterward that he was one of the few in France who maintained his post when the plague hit, and this pattern was repeated across the continent.

With doctors hurrying away from plague victims, it then fell to others to care for them. Many of those who stepped into the breach were members of religious orders. Across Europe desperate patients made their way to monasteries and convents in hopes that the monks or nuns could offer something to ease the pain. Monks sometimes ventured into the homes of the sick to do what they could, and some nuns worked tirelessly in hospitals. Religious orders were no more able than the doctors to cure the plague, but they could and did help by cleaning the patients after they vomited, holding their hands through the worst of the coughing, and generally offering sympathy and comfort. At one Paris hospital, for example, nuns were widely applauded for their work with plague victims. "The saintly sisters," wrote one commentator, "worked sweetly and with great humility, setting aside consideration of earthy dignity."[44]

To be fair to those who avoided working with the sick, the Black Death was highly contagious. Any doctor, monk, or nun who spent significant time among plague patients had a heightened chance of catching the disease as well. De Chauliac, the physician who called out his colleagues for evading their duties, understood the danger; he reported

The medieval Roman Catholic Church included two main groups. One was the laity, or the ordinary worshippers who played no particular role in services and had no special authority within the church. The other was the clergy, made up of monks, priests, and bishops. These men—and they all were men—were allowed to administer Holy Communion, hear confessions, and carry out other important sacraments. According to church practice, these sacraments could be performed only by the clergy.

This presented a significant issue during the Black Death. As clergymen died of the plague, many parishes were left without anyone to administer the sacraments. In particular, no one was available to offer those who were dying of the plague the sacrament of penance. In church doctrine, penance—in which the dying admitted their sins and were forgiven for them—was essential for the salvation of souls. Those who did not confess could not go to heaven.

To remedy the situation, English bishop Ralph Shrewsbury wrote a directive that dramatically expanded the role of the laity and women. "Persuade all men," Shrewsbury told his priests, "that, if they are on the point of death and cannot secure the services of a priest, then they should make confession to each other . . . or if no man is present, then even to a woman." The change did not last: the privilege of hearing confession was withdrawn from the laity as soon as the crisis had passed.

Quoted in Robert S. Gottfried, *The Black Death*. New York: Macmillan, 1983.

afterward that he was always afraid of catching the illness. The monks and nuns who took care of the sick and dying frequently came down with the plague and often died from it too. At the Paris hospital where the "saintly sisters" had done such compelling work, the chronicler claimed that "a great number . . . were called to new life and now rest, it is piously believed, with Christ."[45]

## Laws, Religion, and the Plague

Recognizing that medicine was unable to stop the Black Death or ease the suffering of the plague victims, government leaders offered solutions of their own. Several European cities passed laws designed to keep the pestilence out. Venice forced incoming ships to anchor off the coast for up to forty days before entering the city's harbor. If the crew showed no sign of the Black Death during this time, Venetian officials allowed them in. City authorities elsewhere prevented citizens who were traveling in plague-ridden areas from returning home or required the coffins of plague victims to be nailed down lest the contagion escape. These measures made some sense, but they were difficult to enforce and did little to keep out the rats and fleas that were the primary carriers of the disease.

Religious leaders were active in plague prevention as well. To the people of medieval Europe, God was not a distant, uninvolved figure but a potent force in everyday life. According to the theology of the time, whatever happened on the earth was God's will. Moreover, God's general attitude toward his people could be divined by examining earthly events. An abundant harvest or a military victory signaled God's approval, while droughts or earthquakes were signs of God's displeasure. Priests, bishops, and ordinary Europeans alike spent much

*A member of the clergy comforts people sickened by the plague. Monks, nuns, and some other members of the clergy tried to help those afflicted by illness but they could do little more than offer sympathy and comfort as the plague ravaged cities and towns all across Europe.*

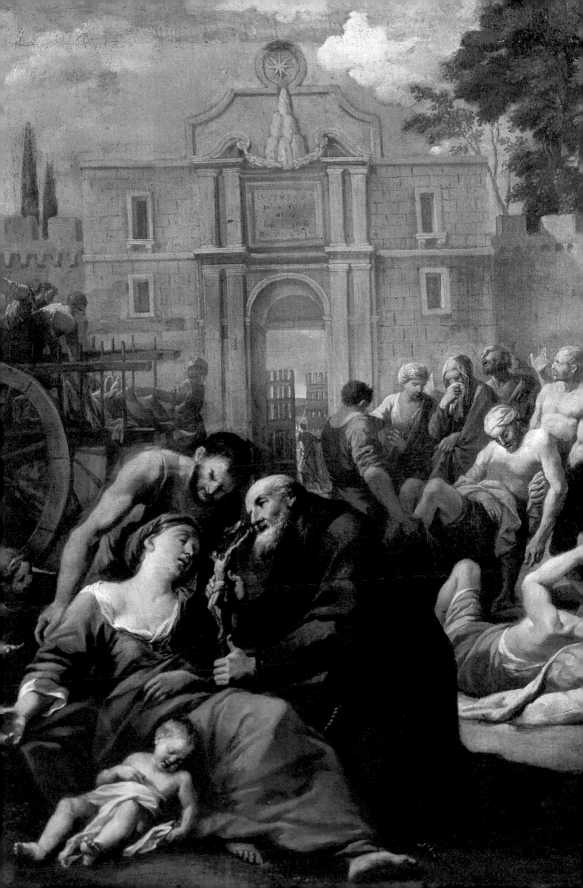

time and energy trying to determine God's feelings as revealed in the events around them.

Not surprisingly, the people of the Middle Ages viewed the plague as a symbol of God's extreme anger at humanity. As de Mussis wrote, "[God] looked down from heaven and saw the entire human race wallowing in a mire of manifold wickedness, enmeshed in wrongdoing, pursuing numberless vices . . . and chasing after everything evil."[46] It was a serious charge against humanity, but one widely accepted among Europeans of the time. If people had been behaving as they should, they wondered, why would God have allowed the plague to cause such devastation? "Plague is killing men," wrote a poet of the period, "because vices rule unchallenged here."[47]

## Public Confession and Gifts to Charity

If God had brought the plague in response to human cruelty and sinfulness, then the only way to stop the epidemic was to get humanity back into God's favor. Accordingly, religious leaders, often supported by government authorities, stepped in to do just that. In Rouen, France, leaders banned drinking, gambling, and a host of other possibly sinful behaviors in hopes of mollifying God's wrath. In Siena, Italy, authorities donated a thousand gold pieces to the poor in an attempt to convince God that they had repented of earlier sins. Pope Clement authorized gatherings in which hundreds of people marched in procession for up to three days, publicly confessing their sins and praying for mercy. Many covered themselves in ashes and dressed in coarse, scratchy clothing to show their willingness to mend their ways.

Despite the gifts to charity, the mass displays of contrition, and the banning of sinful behavior, the religious responses of medieval Europeans—like the medical and governmental attempts—had little discernible impact on the Black Death. The plague did not come to an abrupt end because the people of Siena remembered to help the poor, nor did public confessions convince God to step in and heal the sick. Indeed, some of the solutions offered by the religious establishment actually caused harm. Gathering hundreds of penitents together for a massive display of piety, whatever else it may have accomplished, provided a prime opportunity for the Black Death to spread even further.

Nonetheless, the medical, governmental, and religious authorities who desperately sought a solution to the plague should not be judged too harshly. They took their duties seriously, and they did what they thought best under the difficult circumstances the Black Death presented. Given the enemy they were up against, together with the lack of scientific understanding of the time, it is difficult to see what more these men and women could have done. Faced with a catastrophe so large, so sweeping, and so far beyond the experience of anyone living at the close of the Middle Ages, those who stepped up and fought the pestilence deserve credit for daring to respond at all.

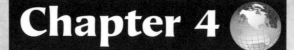

# Chapter 4

# Terror, Despair, and the End of the World

From 1347 to 1351, the Black Death was constantly at the forefront of Europe's attention. From Spain to Russia and from Greece to Iceland, the people of Europe spent their time and energy focused on the Black Death. If the infection had not yet come to their part of the continent, they worried about its arrival. If the plague were raging through their region, they could think only of the death and sorrow that surrounded them. And once the plague had passed through their communities, the Black Death remained uppermost in people's minds as they tried to come to terms with the damage left in its wake. It was a time of terror, sorrow, and despair, and the responses of people to the plague were grounded in these emotions.

## Fear and the Plague's Arrival

For most Europeans, fear and alarm arrived soon after the plague appeared on their continent. In general, word of the plague traveled well in advance of the disease itself. Though the Black Death struck Sicily in the fall of 1347 and reached coastal Italy shortly afterward, for example, it did not attack northern Europe until the following summer. In the interim, however, rumors of the plague's effects in Italy drifted northward. By the spring of 1348 northern Europeans were very aware of what was happening along the Mediterranean. This pattern repeated itself again and again as the plague spread. Except for the people of Messina, who were taken completely by surprise when the infection appeared in their harbor, Europeans who suffered through the pestilence knew in advance that it was coming.

This was a terrifying thought. People who had seen the plague, after all, described it in unrelievedly awful terms: the cries of the dying, the piles of bodies, the loss of loved ones. Moreover, neither medicine, nor prayer, nor laws had stemmed the contagion. It seemed inevitable to most Europeans that the pestilence would eventually reach their homelands too, and waiting for the disease to strike was excruciating. "Everyone in our neighborhood, all of us, everyone in Paris is frightened,"[48] wrote a Parisian shortly before the Black Death finally arrived in 1348.

The fear only intensified as the Black Death moved closer. In towns across Europe, people barricaded themselves in their homes in an effort to avoid infection. Even before the first recorded death in a community, the streets became unnaturally quiet as villagers and townspeople stayed indoors. In France, businesses closed as the plague approached; towns throughout Italy saw enormous drops in business transactions preceding outbreaks of the pestilence. No one knew who might be carrying the plague, so it made sense not to associate with anyone. The nearer the Black Death approached, the more people secluded themselves from the rest of the world.

Once the plague struck a community, the situation became even worse. With death no longer simply a threat but a reality, terror reigned. In much of Europe church bells were traditionally rung to announce deaths, but the practice had to be stopped: the constant ringing of the bells as more and more people succumbed to the Black Death, wrote one chronicler, caused "the whole population of the city, men and women alike . . . to be filled with fear."[49] And if townspeople had isolated themselves from others in the days before the plague arrived, they did so even more zealously now. Many would not even touch objects that had belonged to other people for fear of contamination.

## The Social Contract

This every-man-for-himself attitude became increasingly common as time passed. In many places the social contract began to break down altogether. Instead of following the biblical injunction to "love thy neighbor as thyself" (Mark 12:31), people retreated from others. For many people, self-preservation became more important than any ties binding them to their fellow citizens. "People cared only for their own health,"[50] noted a visitor to Avignon. Gravediggers, priests, and others refused to deal with the dead, terrified that they would catch the pestilence from the corpses. "None could be found to bury the dead for money or friendship,"[51] wrote Agnolo di Tura of Siena, Italy.

Self-preservation showed itself perhaps most obviously in the number of people who ran away from the epidemic. The annals of the plague years include dozens of stories about people who fled their homes as the pestilence approached or after it was active in their communities. Given the Black Death's reach and power, running from the disease was a reasonable reaction to the approaching disaster. Cures and other preventative measures were ineffective, so it did not pay for the people of Europe to sit idly by as the plague swirled around them. Those who ran away were following historical precedent, too: in 1347, after all, hundreds of Messina's residents had poured out of town in search of a safe haven.

As the plague spread, that pattern continued. A wave of people abandoned Venice when the Black Death appeared, most of them hurrying toward Italy's interior, where the epidemic had not yet arrived. Avignon, France, emptied out soon after the plague reached the community in early 1348. In England, Bishop Ralph Shrewsbury opted to leave the congestion—and contagion—of the city for his more isolated estate in the country. King Edward III of England left London while

*The sights and sounds of death were everywhere as the dying cried out for relief and the dead lay in piles awaiting burial. Those who seemed to have escaped the plague's reach waited fearfully or abandoned their friends and loved ones by fleeing.*

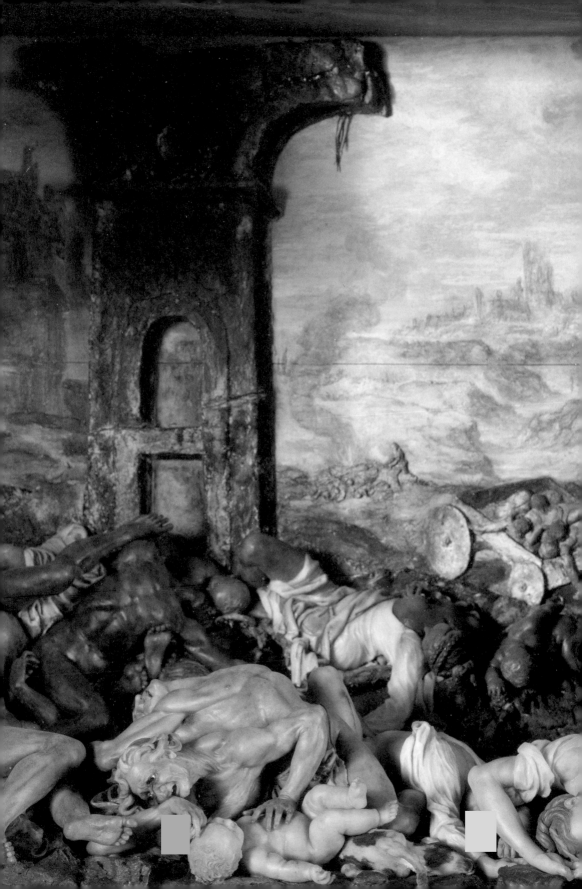

# "One Enormous Joke"

Some Europeans coped with the plague by rejecting any sense of detachment and opted instead for indulgence. According to Giovanni Boccaccio, some of his fellow Italians chose to "drink heavily, enjoy life to the full, go round singing and merrymaking, gratify all of [their] cravings whenever the opportunity offered, and shrug the whole thing off as one enormous joke." For these people, Boccaccio noted, even funerals became an opportunity for laughter.

While recognizing why people were tempted to choose this path, Boccaccio nevertheless did not approve of it. He viewed this behavior as self-indulgent materialism that simply served to distract people from the sad realities of a plague-ridden world. Indeed, Boccaccio believed, behind the jollity, those who gave in to these temptations had more or less given up on life. "People behaved as though their days were numbered," he wrote, "and treated their belongings and their own persons with equal abandon."

Quoted in John Aberth, *From the Brink of Apocalypse.* New York: Routledge, 2000, p. 152.

the plague was at its most active, preferring to spend his time at a rural palace and refusing to reenter the city even for the next session of Parliament a few months later.

Some of the people who fled their homes were accused of cowardice by their neighbors. Others became the targets of wrath, especially if they had used their wealth and social status to escape when other people could not. Shrewsbury was one example. After months of what one chronicler described as "death and death and death"[52] in the towns and villages of his diocese, the bishop emerged from his rural hideaway when the plague showed signs of moving on. Villagers in one local community, however, were incensed to see that the bishop looked rested, well fed, and healthy. Some of them were so angry that they disrupted a church service where Shrewsbury was officiating. Assaulting his attendants, they seized the bishop and held him prisoner overnight.

## Abandoning Family

For most who ran off, though, public disapproval—assuming there was any at all—was short-lived. Even people who did not choose to flee the pestilence, or who did not have the resources to do so, could nevertheless understand why someone else might decide to leave. As Italian author Giovanni Boccaccio pointed out, "against plagues no medicine was better than or even equal to simple flight."[53] Some of the Europeans who ran away, though, received a much less tolerant response from the general public. These were the people who abandoned sick friends and relatives in their haste to get out of town.

There are many references to this practice in contemporary accounts, and all chroniclers who mention it point out that abandoning loved ones was inhuman, appalling, and cruel. "Mother, where have you gone?" Italian chronicler Gabriele de Mussis wrote, supposedly recording the words of a desperately ill child whose mother had left town. "Why are you now so cruel to me when only yesterday you were so kind?"[54] Several sources described the reverse situation—in which grown children left their ill parents—or wrote about situations in which the healthy half of a married couple abandoned the other. "[Sick] relatives were cared for not otherwise than dogs," one writer charged, indicting all runaway family members at once. "They threw them their food and drink by the bed, and then they fled the household."[55]

Not all medieval Europeans, by any means, abandoned their ill friends and families. In plenty of cases family members loyally stood by one another until death. Often the loyalty continued into the grave, as people made sure their loved ones were given a proper burial. "And I," wrote Agnolo di Tura, "buried my five children with my own hands, and so did many others likewise."[56] Some ordinary Europeans even took care of people who were not close friends or relatives simply because they recognized that the patients needed help and no one else was providing it. Still, what struck most commentators was not the number of people who discharged their duties or risked their lives to be helpful but the number who saved their own skins at the expense of others.

Just as Europeans' treatment of friends, family, and neighbors deteriorated during the plague years, their treatment of strangers worsened as well. Fearing that travelers might bring in the plague, Venice blocked outsiders from entering the city limits. The entire kingdom of Poland likewise closed its borders. Everywhere, travelers were looked at with suspicion and told to move on quickly. This was particularly true if the traveler was known to come from a plague-ridden community. "The Messinese were so loathed and feared [in Catania] that no man would speak with them," reported one writer, "but hastily fled at the sight of them, holding his breath."[57] But every unknown traveler was subject to the same scrutiny.

## Blaming the Jews

The most intense hostility directed at outsiders during the plague years, however, was that focused by Christian Europeans on the continent's Jews. Though western Europe was overwhelmingly Christian, pockets of Jews had lived in various areas for as long as anyone could remember. In some places they were tolerated by the government, although they seldom enjoyed all the rights and privileges granted to their Christian neighbors. Elsewhere, though, Jews lived a precarious existence, frequently terrorized by Christian citizens and Christian government officials alike.

At some point soon after the Black Death arrived in western Europe, an odd and troubling rumor began to float across the con-

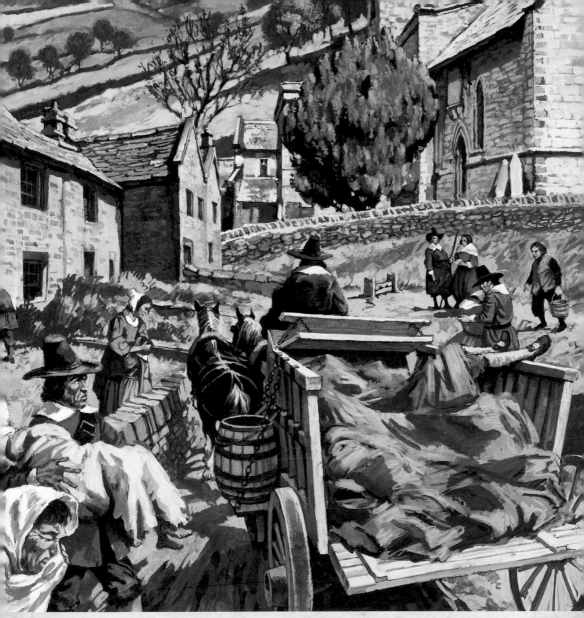

*During an outbreak of bubonic plague in seventeenth-century England, plague victims are taken to a churchyard for burial. While many of the dead were abandoned to the elements, others were buried by grieving family members.*

tinent. The pestilence, people whispered, was not caused by earthquakes, deadly vapors, or the wrath of God; instead, it was the fault of the Jews. In particular, Christians began to charge that Jews were poisoning the wells from which communities obtained their

# The Flagellants

The persecution of the Jews was led in large part, especially in central Europe, by a bizarre movement whose members were known as flagellants. Originally an outgrowth of the mass confessions sponsored by church leaders, the movement took public penance and self-humiliation to extremes. Participants marched through their communities, beating themselves with metal hooks while townspeople watched. "They beat and whipped their bare skin," reported a German chronicler, "until their bodies were bruised and swollen and blood rained down, spattering the walls nearby. . . . Sometimes those bits of metal penetrated the flesh so deeply that it took more than two attempts to pull them out." As they tormented themselves, they begged God for mercy.

Though they originally blamed the plague on their own sinful behavior, the flagellants soon changed tack. By mid-1348 they were enthusiastically blaming the Jews and helping to stir up violence against them. The movement began to disappear only when it started challenging the authority of the Roman Catholic Church, whereupon the pope threatened the arrest of some of the leaders, and the flagellants disbanded. "They disappeared as suddenly as they had come," wrote the chronicler, "as apparitions or ghosts are routed [driven away] by mockery." The damage, however, had been done.

Quoted in Rosemary Horrox, *The Black Death*. New York: Manchester University Press, 1994, pp. 150, 153.

drinking water. The poisoning, of course, was done secretly so no Christians would know. People who drank the tainted water, these rumors alleged, would develop the symptoms of the Black Death and die within days.

Christians of the time should have realized right away that this charge was not only baseless but ridiculous. There were too few Jews to infect all the wells from Norway to Spain and from Ireland to Russia. Nor had a single poisoner been caught in the act. Moreover, Jews contracted the plague—and died from it—at rates comparable to Christians of the period. If the Jews were actually poisoning wells, then, they were forgetting to inform each other. But these facts seemed to escape many of the Christians of the period. Their mood turned uglier than usual, and attacks on Jews began to increase.

A handful of leaders did stop long enough to question the conventional wisdom. Among these was Pope Clement; in 1348 he issued two sharp statements debunking the notion that the wells had been poisoned and instructing Christians to leave the Jews alone. King Casimir of Poland provided protection for the Jews of his kingdom; professors of the medical school in Montpellier, France, likewise argued that all the charges were false. In an ordinary time, these authority figures might have been able to restore sanity in Europe. But the Black Death was far from an ordinary time, and these reasonable voices were largely ignored.

## Mass Killings

Instead, the rumors grew louder and more insistent. In Belgium and Germany, Switzerland and France, Christian mobs—and often Christian government officials as well—were only too happy to blame Jews for the Black Death. Convinced against all evidence to the contrary that their theories were accurate, they set out to manufacture proof by torturing suspected poisoners. At some point during the ordeal, unable to bear the pain any longer, many of the accused offered false confessions. "They had bred spiders and toads in pots and pans," a monk noted, summarizing some of these confessions, "and had obtained poison from overseas." The torture also revealed how Jewish leaders had kept the poisonings a secret for so long. "Not every Jew knew about this wickedness," the monk explained, "only the most powerful ones, so that [the secret] would not be betrayed."[58]

Beating a confession out of Jews was not enough for many of Europe's Christians. Across much of the continent, mobs and civic leaders destroyed the property of Jews, forced them to leave town, or put them to death. In April 1348 angry townspeople in Toulon, France, rounded up most of the community's Jews and murdered them. In Strasbourg, France, the following winter, the town council ordered the arrest and execution of all two thousand local Jews. In Belgium, Germany, and Switzerland, Jews were arrested and sentenced to die. The Jewish population of Europe plummeted as the violence spread from one community to another. By one estimate, sixty major Jewish communities across the continent completely vanished. In France, a Jewish man returned home from a trip to discover that his family had been killed and his neighborhood deserted. "There is no one left but me," he wrote. "I sat down and wept in the bitterness of my soul."[59]

Not all of the terror directed at Europe's Jews during the 1340s was sparked by rumors about the cause of the Black Death. Hatred and distrust of Jews was widespread throughout the medieval period, and long before the arrival of the plague it had often degenerated into violent attacks on individual men and women. Even so, the level of viciousness against Jews during the plague years was much more pervasive, much better organized, and much more horrifying than the events of previous decades—and the Black Death was largely to blame. With their world seemingly crumbling all around them, Christians directed their anger at the most vulnerable people in their midst. "Overwhelmed by what was probably the greatest natural calamity ever to strike [their] continent," wrote twentieth-century commentator Philip Ziegler, "[Europeans] reacted by seeking to rival the cruelty of nature in the hideousness of [their] own man-made atrocities."[60]

## "The End of the World"

The abandonment of children, the suspicion of strangers, the violence against the Jews—all of these were signs that the social order of medieval Europe was failing. Certainly the constant fear and sadness served to leach the emotion out of many Europeans. People became numbed by the devastation that surrounded them. The ties that connected people to one another seemed to be vanishing, and people acknowledged neither the delights nor the burdens of life. "In these days was burying

*Blamed for the outbreak of plague, Jews in the German city of Cologne were burned alive in 1349—a scene depicted in this reproduction from a 1493 woodcut. In the absence of an explanation for the horrors of the Black Death, Europe's Christians blamed the plague on the Jews.*

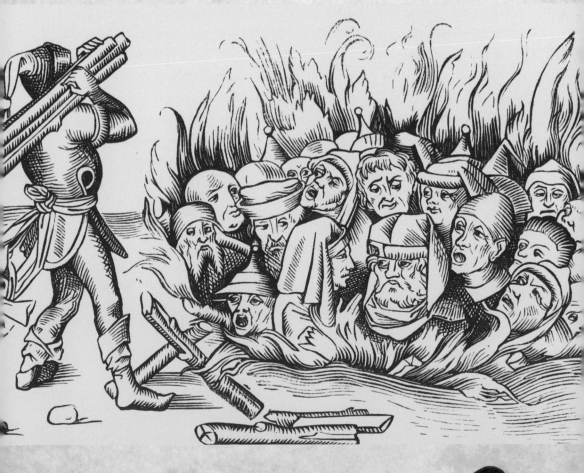

without sorrowe and wedding without friendschippe,"[61] one chronicler observed.

At least some Europeans went through the motions of making lives for themselves. Others retreated into a cocoon of helplessness, doing as little as possible and leading some observers to believe that they were simply waiting for death to overtake them. "No one had any inclination to concern themselves about the future," wrote a German chronicler, noting that farmers were paying little attention to the chores necessary for their survival. Instead of tending their crops or feeding farm animals, he charged, they "wandered around as if mad."[62]

Then again, many late medieval Europeans fully expected that the Black Death would kill not only themselves but very likely everyone on the earth as well. Any number of commentators, especially within the first year of the plague's arrival in Europe, argued that the pestilence would eliminate all human life. "People said and believed, 'This is the end of the world,'"[63] reported Agnolo di Tura. In Ireland, a monk named John Clynn watched all his monastery brothers sicken and die of the Black Death. Clynn was convinced that the plague would kill him too, which it did. Before his death, however, he appended a note to the chronicle he was writing, a note intended for future generations, if such existed. "I leave parchment for continuing the work," he wrote, "in case anyone should still be alive in the future and any son of Adam can escape this pestilence."[64]

And as many others saw it, even if the Black Death did not represent the literal end of the world, it did mark the end of a way of life. Survivors all across the continent found themselves starting over. Their families were dead, their villages vanished. They had seen the overwhelming suffering of friends and relatives, suffering that could not be eased by prayer, by medicine, or by anything else known to humankind. They had waited in terror for the pestilence to arrive in their part of Europe; they had seen the corpses piled five and six high outside cemetery walls; they had smelled the stench of the sick and heard the wails of the dying. They had watched as commerce ground to a halt, as armed soldiers kept strangers from entering towns, as people beat and killed innocent Jews. "It is impossible for the human tongue to recount the awful truth [of the plague],"[65] wrote Agnolo di Tura, and many survivors would certainly have agreed.

In the years of the Black Death, then, Europeans responded to the plague in a variety of ways. Though the reactions differed, they were sparked by similar experiences, emotions, and realities. The people of western Europe had seen the worst that nature had to offer—and the worst that humanity could offer as well. The world was not the same place any longer, and never would be again, and every European who survived the Black Death knew it.

# Chapter 5

# What Was the Legacy of the Black Death?

**B**y 1352 the Black Death was essentially gone from Europe. Quite simply, *Y. pestis* had run out of potential victims. It had spread across the whole continent, leaving almost no region unscathed. To be sure, Europe was not done with the plague forever. In 1361 it returned briefly, then again in 1369, and again at irregular intervals for the next few centuries. Though many of these outbreaks killed large numbers of people, none resulted in anywhere near the number of fatalities caused by the Black Death; and unlike the Black Death, most were restricted to certain geographic regions. Difficult as these later epidemics were, they did not cause the widespread devastation and loss associated with the Black Death.

With the plague unofficially at an end, Europeans tried to put the disaster behind them and move on. This was no easy task. Given that Europe had lost at least one third of its population in a very short time, Europe's traditional social, economic, and political structures no longer functioned as they once had. Villages sat deserted in the wake of the plague. Fewer farmers were left to work the fields; fewer lords remained to oversee them. Trade routes had been disrupted. Respect for religious leaders diminished during the plague years as priests and bishops proved incapable of putting a stop to the disease. Every medieval institution was affected and changed by the Black Death. Few could ultimately be rebuilt as they had been before the plague arrived. Instead, they were turned into something new.

# Depopulation

Of all the changes the Black Death brought to Europe, the most obvious resulted from the shockingly high death rates across the continent. Losing up to half the continent's population left an enormous hole in daily life. With many merchants and notaries dead, even simple business transactions were delayed for weeks or months. Government leaders who died in the plague included King Alfonso XI of Castile (today part of Spain), and Joan the Lame, queen of France, along with countless mayors and town councilmen. Priests were hard hit too: "The contagious pestilence," wrote one observer, "has left many parish churches . . . without an incumbent, so that their inhabitants are bereft of a priest."[66] Europe was in desperate need of political stability and knowledgeable leadership, but too many of its most capable and qualified leaders were no longer alive.

Perhaps the greatest problems, however, lay in agriculture. A typical manor in the postplague period had just lost a third to a half of its workforce. Peasants were already worked to the limit, so it was impossible for them to do the work of those who had died in addition to carrying out their own duties. Thus, in the years after the plague, farmers could not produce large harvests. An English cleric described the scene on a manor left without a full complement of workers. "Crops rotted unharvested in the fields," he wrote. "Livestock wandered around without a shepherd."[67]

Because there were many fewer people to feed than there had been just a few years earlier, the reduced crop yield of the early 1350s did not necessarily represent an enormous problem in itself. The farms did not need to produce as much grain, meat, and dairy as they had before the arrival of the pestilence. But death rates varied by region, and in some places the rate at which farmers died was above the rate for those in towns and cities. In these regions, a smaller food supply did mean that people went hungry. The problem was also more significant in places where great effort was needed to keep fields under cultivation. Some low-lying farmland in the Netherlands, for example, had been reclaimed from the ocean many years earlier and was now protected from the sea by artificial dikes. With so many peasants dead of the plague, though, some Dutch communities could no longer keep the dikes properly maintained. These dikes burst, flooding and destroying valuable acres of farmland.

Commerce suffered too. Numerous cities and nations had stopped trading with each other as the plague spread. Even if traders had wanted to keep doing business, and many did, commerce necessarily came to a halt when governments closed ports and kept outsiders from coming in. At the same time, the deaths of millions of farmers, loggers, weavers, and carpenters caused production of goods such as cloth, lumber, and wool to decline considerably. Even the most dedicated merchants, then, could not easily obtain materials for trade. In the wake of the plague, the mercantile progress Europeans had made during the previous century largely vanished.

## Resiliency

To many Europeans in the years following the Black Death, the challenges of making the world run again seemed completely overwhelming. They faced declining commerce, churches without priests, and governments without leaders. For some, life seemed downright impossible. English chronicler Thomas Walsingham, for example, wrote that "the world could never again regain its former prosperity."[68] Giovanni Boccaccio agreed, though he focused on the decline of morality. "The public distress was such that all laws, whether human or divine, were ignored,"[69] he complained at one point. The damage caused by the plague, these thinkers feared, might prove too great for civilization to be rebuilt.

But Europeans were more resilient than Walsingham and Boccaccio guessed. "Life did go on," writes historian Chris Given-Wilson, "and the irony is that for most of those who survived . . . it got better."[70] The main reason for the improvement was both paradoxical and ghoulish: The depopulation of Europe in the Black Death indirectly made it a healthier place. Before the plague, historians agree, the population of Europe outstripped the food supply. To meet the demand for grain, farmers were forced to cultivate more and more land, much of it

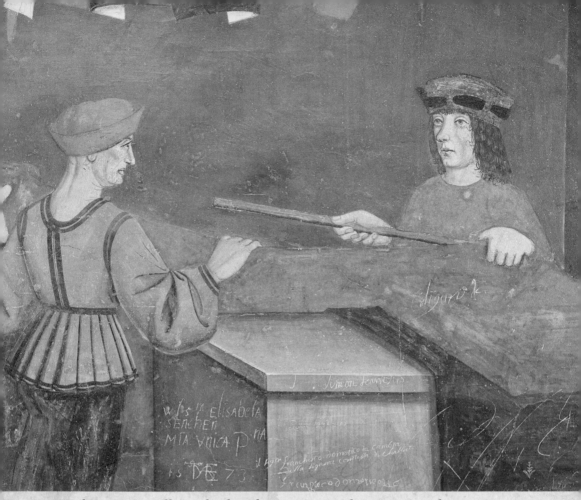

*With so many millions dead and governments closing ports to keep outsiders away, cloth merchants (pictured) and other businessmen and women had difficulty obtaining materials for trade. Regional economies suffered, as did the finances of individuals and families.*

less than ideal for growing crops. "Agriculture was being pushed to the margin," notes a modern source, "where the effort of production was often greater than the output."[71] Even in good years, many people were constantly hungry.

Reducing Europe's population by a third eased a great deal of the pressure on farmers. Once they were back on the job, a process that admittedly took several years after the end of the Black Death, they did not need to plant grain in marginal lands. With only the best land in production, the same amount of work produced an almost equally good harvest. The smaller postplague population could

# Backlash

In the years following the plague, governments and employers grew increasingly concerned that the chronic labor shortage gave workers too much power. Several countries passed laws designed to limit what laborers could earn and where they could work, but these laws were often ignored. A petition to England's Parliament in 1376 summed up the employers' perspective:

> Although various ordinances and statues have been made in several parliaments to punish labourers, artificers [craftsmen] and other servants, yet these have continued subtly and by great malice aforethought, to escape the penalty of the said ordinances and statutes. As soon as their masters accuse them of bad service, or wish to pay them for their labour according to the form of the statutes [that is, pay them at preplague rates], they take flight and suddenly leave their employment and district . . . for they are taken into service immediately in new places, at such dear wages that example and encouragement is afforded to all servants to depart into fresh places, and go from master to master as soon as they are displeased about any matter. For fear of such flight, [employers] now dare not challenge or offend their servants, but give them whatever they wish to ask, in spite of the statutes and ordinances to the contrary.

Quoted in John Aberth, *From the Brink of Apocalypse*. New York: Routledge, 2000, p. 136.

not completely stop starvation, of course; even with millions fewer mouths to feed, a summer of bad weather could still destroy crops and lead to famine. But the records show that starvation became less common following the Black Death's disappearance from Europe. For the first time in years, the land could actually produce enough food to sustain life.

## Worker and Employer

The smaller population had several other beneficial effects on farmers as well. Most significantly, as the population dropped, the power of the individual farmer rose. Under feudalism, the fundamental political and economic system of the medieval period, most peasants were serfs. These tenant farmers cultivated land belonging to lords and paid rent to the landowners in the form of a share of the grain they produced. Laws usually barred serfs from moving to another manor; peasants in feudal society belonged to the land and, by extension, to the lord who owned it. There could be no competition for laborers, then, however strong or efficient. "For the lord who held the land," writes historian Robert S. Gottfried, "the century after 1250 [that is, up until the Black Death] was an era of economic prosperity; for the peasants who worked it, it was an era of unqualified disaster."[72]

In the years after the Black Death, though, the traditional labor glut on European farms suddenly became a labor shortage. For the first time in generations, landowning nobles needed more farmworkers than they had. Tenants realized that they did not have to stay on the manor of their birth; they had options, in reality if not always in law. With every landowner dealing with a reduced number of serfs, competition for the survivors became intense. Some lords offered lower rents in hopes of attracting more farmers to move to their property, in some cases trimming rents to nothing. "Better no revenue at all," writes historian Barbara Tuchman, looking at the matter from the perspective of the landowner, "than that cleared land should be retaken by wilderness."[73]

Costs fell following the Black Death, too, which was likewise to the benefit of peasants. "There were small prices for virtually everything," wrote English chronicler Henry Knighton. "A man could have a horse, which was [previously] worth 40 shillings, for 6 shillings 8 pence, a cow for 12 pence."[74] Combined with the lower rents, the reduced cost of living helped many European peasants live much more comfortably after the Black Death than they had before it. Peasants did not become rich by any means, and life for most was still precarious; at best, they went from being extremely poor to being merely very poor. Still, it is clear that depopulation associated with the Black Death changed the circumstances of the peasants for the better.

## From Feudalism Toward Capitalism

Indeed, many historians credit the Black Death with hastening the downfall of feudalism. Even under the feudal system, larger manors often housed a group of men known as day laborers. Unlike ordinary serfs, who had a particular plot of land to cultivate, these men moved from one farm to another, assisting with plowing, harvesting, or other agricultural tasks as needed. They produced no crops of their own, so landowners paid them directly for their work. Through most of the medieval era, the payment was barely enough to live on; the serfs of the time, even with their crushing rents, usually did better than the day laborers.

But in the wake of the Black Death, wages for day laborers skyrocketed. In one notable example, English farmhands who earned two shillings a week in 1347 saw their pay jump to more than ten shillings a week in 1350. It was much more possible to earn a decent living with wages like these, and more and more peasants began to see working for wages as a better and more dignified option than laboring for months to produce a crop, most of which would go to the landlord. As a result, peasants increasingly chose to become independent workers. "Serfdom, in decline before the mortality, now disappeared entirely," writes historian John Kelly. "A man could simply up and leave a manor, secure in the knowledge that wherever he settled, someone would hire him."[75]

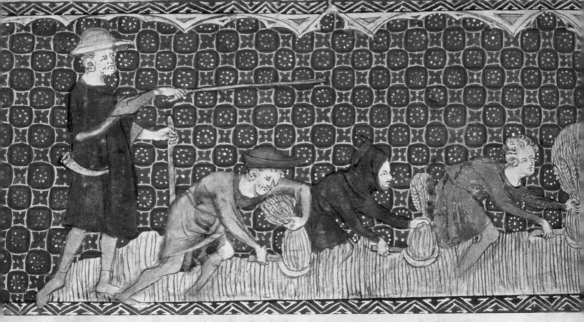

*As the shadow of death receded, landowners were faced with shortages of serfs who could sow seeds and harvest crops. Little by little the labor shortage led to higher wages and better working and living conditions for peasant farmers (pictured).*

Following the Black Death, then, feudalism gave way to the beginnings of a capitalist economy, one based on cash rather than on land, wages rather than barter, and short-term contracts rather than lifetime legal obligations.

The increase in the standard of living of European peasants following the plague applied to other workers as well. The death toll of the plague had created labor shortages everywhere, not just on the farm, and the poor took advantage by demanding better pay. "Serving girls," Italian writer Matteo Villani complained, "want at least 12 florins per year and the more arrogant among them 18 or 24 florins." The changes were even more obvious in the case of skilled craftsmen. Even before the Black Death, employers had a limited pool of potential workers to draw from to fill the posts of weavers, clerks, and other jobs that required significant training. After the pestilence, demand soared, and workers received enormous pay raises. "Minor artisans working with their hands want three times . . . the usual pay,"[76] Villani sniffed.

The increase in wages soon produced a backlash not just among the Villanis of the world but among government leaders as well. In an

## Death and Art

The Black Death was a trauma unlike anything the people of the time had ever experienced, and the scars it produced were everywhere. Sometimes these scars were visible. Deserted villages and overflowing cemeteries, for example, symbolized the massive death toll of the plague years and continued to do so for many years afterward. But these scars could be invisible as well, living on in the emotions and thoughts of the survivors and being expressed indirectly through their actions.

The art of the postplague world, for example, clearly shows how people of the era thought about death. In earlier art, points out historian Barbara Tuchman, death was frequently personified as a skeleton, but in the 1350s and 1360s that began to change. One painting of the period, for example, shows death as "a black-cloaked old woman with streaming hair and wild eyes, carrying a broad-bladed murderous scythe. Her feet end in claws instead of toes." Another artwork from the time shows grotesque corpses confronting a group of living men and women. "In their silks and curls and fashionable hats," writes Tuchman, "the party of vital handsome men and women stare appalled at what they will become." Death, the artwork of the time remind viewers, awaits us all—and it will be by no means a pleasant, sanitized experience.

Barbara Tuchman, *A Distant Mirror: The Calamitous Fourteenth Century.* New York: Alfred A. Knopf, 1978, pp. 124–25.

effort to restore the traditional balance between workers and employers, the king of England issued a decree forcing laborers and artisans to accept whatever jobs they were offered at the salaries they had received before the plague. The French government passed a similar law, though this one did allow workers a small wage increase. The laws were not notably successful, as market forces proved more powerful than the dictates of kings and councils; many workers refused to follow the laws, and employers often paid well above the official wage scale. A new era had begun. The depopulation caused by the Black Death was changing the European economic system.

## Technology and Medicine

Besides upsetting the balance between worker and employer, the Black Death led to a number of other important changes. Lower population levels, for example, encouraged technological innovation as people learned to do more with less help. New methods of catching fish allowed fishing vessels to fill their holds as quickly as before, even though crews were smaller. New weaving techniques likewise enabled a reduced number of weavers to produce plenty of cloth. Even warfare was affected. With fewer soldiers serving in armies, military strategists designed new, powerful weapons that could make up for the reduced numbers of fighting men. Thus, the depopulation of the Black Death indirectly led to the widespread use of firearms—a development with enormous consequences for the world.

The Black Death also changed the way people thought about medicine. The medical field had not distinguished itself during the epidemic. Too many doctors had run off instead of caring for the sick, and medical techniques of the time had been unable to stop or cure the disease. Following the plague, some physicians realized that their entire profession needed to do better. Over time, medical training became more hands-on and less theoretical, and doctors behaved more like modern scientists. "Rather than deducing a conclusion from pure reason," writes Kelly, the physician in the postplague period "posited a theory, tested the theory against observable fact, and rigorously analyzed the results to see if they supported the theory."[77] In Kelly's view, the changes in medical practices after the Black Death represented the first stirrings of the scientific method.

Governments also realized that they needed to play a greater role in protecting people's health. The Black Death spurred several municipalities to establish special health boards. In Florence, for example, the board was charged with helping to keep the city clean—or at least cleaner than it had been in the past—and prescribing how corpses should be buried to avoid spreading disease. The significance of these health boards is not so much what they accomplished at the time— the state of medical knowledge limited what they could do—but their very existence; they show governments' rising sense of responsibility for keeping communities as disease-free as possible. Later health boards would take ever greater steps to safeguard the health of the community.

## Religion and the Church

The plague had a significant effect on religion as well. Like the medical field, the Roman Catholic Church had not distinguished itself during the Black Death. It had failed to provide answers or cures, and its leaders had often seemed ineffective and remote. Too many priests and bishops had run off instead of caring for the sick and dying; too many clerics of all types had charged enormous fees for assisting those they did help. Unlike physicians, however, church leaders saw nothing wrong with their work. Officials insisted that misconduct on the part of clerics had been extremely rare, and they argued that the fees were justified because the bulk of the money collected was used to help the poor. There may have been some truth to both assertions, but from a public relations standpoint, church officials should probably have responded with more humility. The Christians of western Europe were in no mood to hear how well their church had responded to the disaster when, in their experience, the opposite was true.

In the years after the plague, then, the reputation of the church suffered. At best, many Christians charged that it had drifted away from God. At worst, it was seen as a thoroughly corrupt institution far more interested in enriching itself than in saving souls. Either way, it lost credibility with many Europeans in the wake of the plague. Even the pope recognized the widespread hypocrisy of many clerics. "What can you preach to the people?" he demanded of his bishops in 1351. "If on humility, you yourself are the proudest of the world, pumped up, pompous and sumptuous in luxuries. . . . If on chastity—but we will be

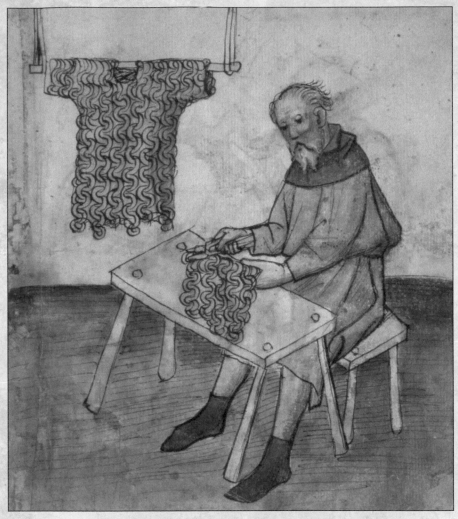

*Because so many of their peers had died from the plague, skilled craftsmen could demand higher pay for their work once the worst of the contagion had passed. Makers of armor (pictured) as well as weavers and others were part of a rebalancing of the European economic system.*

silent on this, for God knoweth what each man does and how many of you satisfy your lusts."[78]

Few Christians of the time, however, dared to reject the church outright. Despite its troubles, the church remained the one road to salvation; renouncing the church meant a sure path to hell. But as dissatisfaction grew, Christians increasingly began clamoring for change. Reform movements sprang up around figures such as John Wycliffe, an English thinker vocal in his disapproval of what the church had become. When the church did not respond as the critics saw fit, the chorus of condemning voices rose. In the early 1500s, under the leadership of German monk Martin Luther, many northern Europeans broke away from the church in what became known as the Protestant Reformation. It would not be accurate to say that the church's reaction to the Black Death caused the Reformation; too many other factors were involved. However, the church's actions during the plague, together with its response to criticisms afterward, undoubtedly helped create conditions allowing the Reformation to take place.

## Legacy

For survivors of the Black Death, the plague represented not one tragedy but two. The first, of course, was the death of so many people: husbands and wives, sons and daughters, siblings and parents—losses in many cases much greater than any person should ever have to bear. But the Black Death also caused another kind of loss: the loss of a world. For all its faults, the world of the early 1300s seemed stable enough. Its patterns and rhythms provided familiarity and comfort. Medical leaders offered cures, priests offered absolution; the feudal system provided a structure for a life of work and assigned people a clear place in the social hierarchy.

The Black Death destroyed that stability. In its place, at first, it seemed to offer survivors of the epidemic nothing of any value—just a weary, lonely, and impoverished existence, haunted by the memories of frenzied flight, overflowing graveyards, and the agonized screams of dying loved ones. But as time went on, the survivors began picking up the pieces of their lives. Recognizing that there was no way back to the world they had once known, they started the process of creating something new.

What they created was not perfect by any means. The postplague world that Europeans built was still skewed toward the rich, still a place of violence and ethnic hatred, still a place where people lived on the margins and hunger was all too common. But the people of the time were taking important steps toward a greater goal: a world where even the common people could enjoy an occasional luxury item, a world where science and technology would take on a new importance, and most of all, perhaps, a world where sickness no longer would hold such power. The courage they showed in beginning the process of constructing such a world is perhaps the greatest legacy of the Black Death.

# Source Notes

**Introduction: The Defining Characteristics
of the Black Death**

1. Quoted in Barbara Tuchman, *A Distant Mirror: The Calamitous Fourteenth Century*. New York: Alfred A. Knopf, 1978, p. 98.
2. Quoted in Joseph P. Byrne, *The Black Death*. Westport, CT: Greenwood, 2004, p. 152.
3. John Aberth, *From the Brink of Apocalypse*. New York: Routledge, 2000, p. 110.
4. Quoted in John Kelly, *The Great Mortality*. New York: HarperCollins, 2005, p. 110.
5. Quoted in Philip Alcabes, *Dread: How Fear and Fantasy Have Fueled Epidemics from the Black Death to Avian Flu*. New York: Public Affairs, 2009, p. 45.
6. Quoted in Tuchman, *A Distant Mirror*, p. 101.
7. Quoted in Aberth, *From the Brink of Apocalypse*, p. 153.
8. Quoted in Kelly, *The Great Mortality*, p. 126.

**Chapter One: What Conditions Led to the Black Death?**

9. Quoted in Aberth, *From the Brink of Apocalypse*, p. 14.
10. Quoted in David Herlihy, *The Black Death and the Transformation of the West*, ed. Samuel K. Cohn Jr. Cambridge, MA: Harvard University Press, 1997, p. 32.
11. Quoted in Kelly, *The Great Mortality*, p. 72.
12. Aberth, *From the Brink of Apocalypse*, p. 113.
13. Quoted in Walter Shaw Sparrow, *Old England: Her Story Mirrored in Her Scenes*. New York: James Pott, 1908, p. 310.
14. Colin Platt, *King Death: The Black Death and Its Aftermath in Late-Medieval England*. Toronto: University of Toronto Press, 1996, p. 34.
15. Kelly, *The Great Mortality*, p. 64.

16. Kelly, *The Great Mortality*, p. 68.

17. Quoted in Kelly, *The Great Mortality*, p. 109.

18. Geoffrey Chaucer, *The Portable Chaucer*, ed. Theodore Morrison. New York: Penguin, 1949.

19. William J. Bernstein, *A Splendid Exchange: How Trade Shaped the World*. New York: Atlantic Monthly Press, 2008, p. 110.

20. Quoted in Tuchman, *A Distant Mirror*, p. 80.

## Chapter Two: The Black Death Arrives

21. Quoted in Kelly, *The Great Mortality*, p. 7.

22. Quoted in Kelly, *The Great Mortality*, p. 34.

23. Quoted in Samuel Anthony Barnett, *The Story of Rats: Their Impact on Us, and Our Impact on Them*. Crows Nest, Australia: Allen and Unwin, 2001, p. 3.

24. Robert Sullivan, *Rats*. New York: Bloomsbury, 2004, p. 137.

25. Bernstein, *A Splendid Exchange*, p. 139.

26. Quoted in Robert S. Gottfried, *The Black Death*. New York: Free Press, 1983, p. 36.

27. Quoted in Bernstein, *A Splendid Exchange*, p. 140.

28. Quoted in Bernstein, *A Splendid Exchange*, p. 142.

29. Quoted in Kelly, *The Great Mortality*, p. 84.

30. Quoted in Aberth, *From the Brink of Apocalypse*, p. 119.

31. Quoted in Kelly, *The Great Mortality*, p. 87.

32. Gottfried, *The Black Death*, p. 42.

33. Kelly, *The Great Mortality*, p. 88.

## Chapter Three: Medicine, Laws, and Prayer

34. Quoted in Aberth, *From the Brink of Apocalypse*, p. 120.

35. Tuchman, *A Distant Mirror*, p. 99.

36. Tuchman, *A Distant Mirror*, p. 105.

37. Kelly, *The Great Mortality*, p. 165.

38. Quoted in Sullivan, *Rats*, p. 139.

39. Quoted in Tuchman, *A Distant Mirror*, p. 106.

40. Quoted in Gottfried, *The Black Death*, p. 112.

41. Quoted in Gottfried, *The Black Death*, p. 116.

42. Kelly, *The Great Mortality*, p. 171.

43. Quoted in Aberth, *From the Brink of Apocalypse*, p. 119.

44. Quoted in Kelly, *The Great Mortality*, p. 180.

45. Quoted in Kelly, *The Great Mortality*, p. 180.

46. Quoted in Aberth, *From the Brink of Apocalypse*, p. 114.

47. Quoted in Sullivan, *Rats*, p. 141.

**Chapter Four: Terror, Despair, and the End of the World**

48. Quoted in Kelly, *The Great Mortality*, p. 176.

49. Quoted in Gottfried, *The Black Death*, p. 55.

50. Quoted in Herlihy, *The Black Death and the Transformation of the West*, p. 62.

51. Quoted in Gottfried, *The Black Death*, p. 45.

52. Quoted in Kelly, *The Great Mortality*, p. 194.

53. Quoted in Herlihy, *The Black Death and the Transformation of the West*, p. 40.

54. Quoted in Aberth, *From the Brink of Apocalypse*, p. 154.

55. Quoted in Herlihy, *The Black Death and the Transformation of the West*, p. 62.

56. Quoted in Tuchman, *A Distant Mirror*, p. 101.

57. Quoted in Bernstein, *A Splendid Exchange*, p. 142.

58. Quoted in Sullivan, *Rats*, p. 141.

59. Quoted in Kelly, *The Great Mortality*, p. 138.

60. Philip Ziegler, *The Black Death*. New York: Harper and Row, 1969, p. 109.

61. Quoted in Tuchman, *A Distant Mirror*, p. 100.

62. Quoted in Tuchman, *A Distant Mirror*, p. 103.

63. Quoted in Tuchman, *A Distant Mirror*, p. 99.

64. Quoted in Chris Given-Wilson, ed., *An Illustrated History of Late Medieval England*. New York: Manchester University Press, 1996, p. 4.

65. Quoted in Gottfried, *The Black Death*, p. 45.

**Chapter Five: What Was the Legacy of the Black Death?**

66. Quoted in Aberth, *From the Brink of Apocalypse*, pp. 160–61.

67. Quoted in Aberth, *From the Brink of Apocalypse*, p. 132.

68. Quoted in Tuchman, *A Distant Mirror*, p. 103.

69. Quoted in Albert S. Lyons and R. Joseph Petrucelli, *Medicine: An Illustrated History.* New York: Abradale, 1978, p. 349.

70. Given-Wilson, ed., *An Illustrated History of Late Medieval England*, p. 4.

71. UK Agriculture, "UK Countryside History—1300 AD," www.uk agriculture.com.

72. Gottfried, *The Black Death*, p. 26.

73. Tuchman, *A Distant Mirror*, p. 125.

74. Quoted in Gottfried, *The Black Death*, p. 94.

75. Kelly, *The Great Mortality*, p. 285.

76. Quoted in Kelly, *The Great Mortality*, p. 284.

77. Kelly, *The Great Mortality*, pp. 288–89.

78. Quoted in Tuchman, *A Distant Mirror*, p. 129.

# Important People During the Time of the Black Death

**Agnolo di Tura:** A resident of Siena, Italy, whose wife and five children died in the plague; he chronicled the events in Siena.

**Giovanni Boccaccio:** The Italian author of *The Decameron*, a fictional work set in the time of the Black Death; the introduction to *The Decameron* gives a vivid and accurate account of the plague in Florence, Italy.

**Guy de Chauliac:** A French physician and the pope's personal doctor.

**Pope Clement VI:** Pope during the Black Death; opposed the persecution of Jews and tried to get priests and other clergy to pay more attention to the dying.

**Henry Knighton:** An English chronicler whose writings cover the plague years in England.

**Gabriele de Mussis:** An Italian chronicler whose works make many mentions of the plague in Italy and elsewhere.

**Michele da Piazza:** An Italian monk best known for his descriptions of the arrival of the plague in Sicily and its spread to the Italian mainland.

**Ralph Shrewsbury:** The bishop of Bath and Wells in England, who issued directives allowing women and lay church members to hear confession in the absence of priests; was also attacked by parishioners after abandoning city life at the height of the plague.

# For Further Research

## Books

Philip Alcabes, *Dread: How Fear and Fantasy Have Fueled Epidemics from the Black Death to Avian Flu.* New York: Public Affairs: 2009.

Lynne Elliott, *Medieval Medicine and the Plague.* New York: Crabtree, 2009.

Sean Martin, *The Black Death.* New York: Chartwell, 2009.

Don Nardo, *The Black Death.* Farmington Hills, MI: Gale Cengage, 2011.

Faith Wallis, *Medieval Medicine: A Reader.* Toronto: University of Toronto Press, 2010.

John Withington, *Disaster! A History of Earthquakes, Floods, Plagues, and Other Catastrophes.* New York: Skyhorse, 2010.

Adam Woog, *The Late Middle Ages.* San Diego: ReferencePoint, 2012.

Diane Zahler, *The Black Death.* Minneapolis: Twenty-First Century Books, 2009.

## Internet Sources and Websites

BBC History, "British History in Depth: Black Death." (www.bbc.co.uk/history/british/middle_ages/black_01.shtml). This site discusses the plague in Great Britain, focusing especially on how it arrived, how it spread, and how people responded. Includes excerpts from several first-person accounts.

Eyewitness to History, "The Black Death, 1348." (www.eyewitnesstohistory.com/plague.htm). A brief but informative site with basic information about the Black Death in Europe. Includes several quotes from people who lived through the plague.

Jewish History Sourcebook, "The Black Death and the Jews." (www
.fordham.edu/halsall/jewish/1348-jewsblackdeath.asp). Excerpts from
several primary source accounts relating to the persecution of Europe's
Jews during the years of the Black Death, along with basic background
information for the texts.

ABC Science, "On the Trail of the Black Death." (www.abc.net.au
/science/articles/2004/01/22/2857189.htm). An article about the Black
Death, giving information about its progress and impact and comparing
it to other epidemics throughout history.

Medieval Sourcebook, "Boccaccio: The Decameron—Introduction."
(www.fordham.edu/halsall/source/boccacio2.asp). The text of the introduction to Boccaccio's *Decameron*, an eyewitness account of the
Black Death in Florence, Italy.

# Index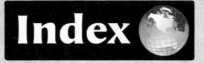

# Picture Credits

Roy 2 B VII f.78 Reaping corn harvest in August, from the Queen Mary Psalter, c.1310-20 (vellum), English School, (14th century)/ British Library, London, UK/© British Library Board. All Rights Reserved/The Bridgeman Art Library: 75

Ms Amb 3172 Armourer Making a Hauberk (pen & ink on paper), German School, (15th century)/Stadtbibliothek, Nuremberg, Germany/The Bridgeman Art Library: 79

# About the Author

Stephen Currie is the author of several dozen books as well as many curriculum materials and magazine articles. His works for ReferencePoint Press include books on the Renaissance, goblins, and hydropower. He has taught at grade levels ranging from kindergarten to college. A native of Chicago, he currently lives in New York State.